Companion Animal Death

CW00952529

*Dedicated to my family, to Jan, and
to all the human and animal friends
who have touched our lives.*

Companion Animal Death

A Practical and Comprehensive Guide for Veterinary Practice

Mary F. Stewart
DVM MRCVS Dip. Couns.
Honorary Senior Research Fellow,
University of Glasgow Veterinary School

Foreword by Colin Murray Parkes OBE MD
FRCPsych.

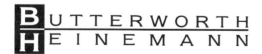

BUTTERWORTH
HEINEMANN

OXFORD AUCKLAND BOSTON JOHANNESBURG MELBOURNE NEW DELHI

Butterworth-Heinemann
Linacre House, Jordan Hill, Oxford OX2 8DP
225 Wildwood Avenue, Woburn, MA 01801-2041
A division of Reed Educational and Professional Publishing Ltd

ℛ A member of the Reed Elsevier plc group

First published 1999

© Reed Educational and Professional Publishing Ltd 1999

British Library Cataloguing in Publication Data
A catalogue record for this book is available from the British Library

Library of Congress Cataloguing in Publication Data
A catalogue record for this book is available from the Library of Congress

ISBN 0 7506 4076 6

Cover photograph by Marty S. Stewart

Typeset by Keyword Typesetting Services Ltd, Wallington, Surrey
Printed and bound in Great Britian by Biddles Ltd, Guildford and King's
Lynn

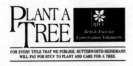

PLANT A TREE
British Trust for Conservation Volunteers
FOR EVERY TITLE THAT WE PUBLISH, BUTTERWORTH-HEINEMANN
WILL PAY FOR BTCV TO PLANT AND CARE FOR A TREE.

Contents

Foreword

It was a balmy day in Elsamere, on the edge of Lake Naivasha. A group of free-living Colubus monkeys had come down from the trees to feed on scraps from the kitchen and I sat quietly watching them until a youngster plucked up the courage to come closer. As he started to take some potato peelings from my hand I gently stroked the back of his arm. The monkey immediately stopped eating, sat back and looked at me. Then he reached forward and gently stroked the back of my arm.

At moments like this the enormous gulf between ourselves and other animals vanishes. We become one species. The experience was moving because it was so unexpected. Yet it is no more surprising than the daily interactions that take place between the companion animals whom we love and who love us. The extraordinary thing is that we take that love for granted.

I use the word love deliberately for I believe that there is no other word that adequately describes the attachment between human beings and their pets. It may seldom be a passionate love in the romantic sense but it is rooted in the same emotional need for closeness that distinguishes it from all other relationships. In fact one can justly say that the sole function of a pet is to love and be loved. That being the case it is hardly surprising if the ending of such relationships by death is a cause for grief.

For many of us the death of a pet is our first bereavement. It will be remembered for the rest of our lives and will colour our attitude to other losses. If it has been well handled we shall be left with the mixture of pain and happiness that is nostalgia. That is certainly how I remember my own first wonderful cat, Timmy, whom I loved with the whole-hearted enthusiasm of a 6-year-old. He died of septicaemia following a rat bite and I remember clearly my mother holding me in her arms as we cried together. It was her love and comfort that mitigated the pain of that loss and helped to prepare me for the other losses that were to come in my life, as they do in the lives of all of us.

In my work as a psychiatrist with a special interest in the effects of grief and loss I have learned that grief is not only a potential threat to physical and mental health, it is also an opportunity for psychological growth. Losses are often turning points in our lives when we are brought up short and forced, unwillingly, to take stock. It sometimes takes a bereavement to teach us the value of the people and other creatures whom we have taken for granted.

Vets and doctors share the privilege and responsibility of being around at such times, and we are often in a position to help people through these painful transitions. Sometimes we may be the only ones who know or care enough to reach out to people who are in desperate need of our support.

Much of the time it is not difficult to prepare people for bereavement and to help them through; all we need to do is to tell them the truth and stay close to them while they cope with its implications. However, there are other times when it can be very hard to do and say the right things. Some people are difficult to help and some situations more traumatic to those who experience them than others. Yet it is these very people who are in greatest need and who are at risk of further problems if we get it wrong.

For these reasons a book such as this is greatly needed and will enable vets to cope with confidence with the losses that they meet in day-to-day veterinary practice. Mary Stewart has pioneered important developments in this field, and her down-to-earth approach and sound advice makes this book an indispensable guide to practice.

Colin Murray Parkes OBE MD FRCPsych.
1 December 1998

Acknowledgements

I would like to express my sincere gratitude to the R.C.V.S. Charter Education Trust for funding a visit to key North American Veterinary Schools, giving me the opportunity to meet and exchange ideas with some of the most progressive thinkers in this area.

Liz Ormerod for her major contribution of researching and supplying material, and for her continual interest.

Those who officially reviewed and in some cases made important contributions to the text:

Terry Daley DIP.COUNS., Wendy McGrandle MRCVS, Liz Ormerod MRCVS, Antony Podberscek MRCVS, Howard Taylor MRCVS, Janet Thomas MRCVS.

Those who have contributed information on special subjects:
Richard Allport MRCVS, Walter Beswick MRCVS RCVS, Nina Bondarenko of Canine Partners for Independence, Janet Ely MRCVS, Ian Fleming MRCVS, David Griffiths and Mandy Jones of Guide Dogs for the Blind Association, April Jones MRCVS and Tania Woods.

John Mould MRCVS and Jill Nicholson who read and commented. Ewan Cameron, Mary Findlay and other staff of Glasgow Vet School, who gave me practical and moral support.

The many people over the years who have directly or indirectly contributed their knowledge of, and enthusiasm for, the subject. Special thanks to those who have been my good friends as well:

Cindy Adams, Sam Ahmedzai, Ron Anderson, Leo Bustad, Mary Bloom, Caroline Butler, Alan Beck, Susan Cohen, Peggy Degraffe, Andrew Edney, Bruce Fogle, James Harris, Lynn Hart, Aaron Katcher, Andrea Le Blanc, Bonnie Madder, David Morton, Roger Mugford, Pete Rogers, Bernie Rollin, Andrew Rowan, Clint Sanders, James Serpell, Cecelia Soares, Vicky Tod and Sally Walshaw.

Anne Docherty, Director of the Society for Companion Animal Studies, and my friend, who believed I could write this book, made sure I did and edited several drafts. Without her, this book would not exist.

Mary F. Stewart

Preface: why is this book needed?

Although, for ease of writing, this book is mostly addressed to veterinary students and practitioners, it is also intended for veterinary nurses and other staff who would like to develop a familiarity and ease with the emotional side of their work, and establish good practices that increase their own and clients' confidence and satisfaction, and that help to ensure the well-being of their patients.

To be a successful practitioner of human or veterinary medicine, it is necessary to develop a 'whole person' understanding of our professional role; it is not just the obvious clinical skills which are involved. As well as being a science, the practice of veterinary medicine is undoubtedly an art and it is that aspect that matters most to the clients.

In general, the veterinary profession has a wonderful reputation. The images presented by the frequent, popular programmes usually imply that most vets are good tempered, even jolly sort of folk, who all care deeply about the animals in their care, and are considerate and supportive of their clients. People often say they wish their doctors were as caring as their vets and that human hospitals treated their patients as sensitively as vet hospitals treat animals.

This leads to a very high expectation of all vets who work with companion animals. We are expected to be comfortable at dealing with all different kinds of animals and their owners, always remaining calm and supportive through all sorts of emotional and situational crises, no matter what else is going on in our own sometimes very stressful lives.

Part of the difficulty starts in the later years of secondary school. British pupils who wish to enter Veterinary School need to make career decisions at a young age. They are required to concentrate on a fairly limited scientific subject matter and it becomes a 'head down', goal-oriented experience. There is not a lot of spare time to explore ideas and widen horizons.

Some of the reasons students choose veterinary science as a career include:

- **Because they like animals.** Being equally qualified for entrance to Medical School, many students choose Veterinary School because they would rather work with animals than with people.
- **Because they do not always know what it involves.** When pupils volunteer to work with a local vet, they usually help 'in the back' where patients are treated and operations done. They do not usually sit in on consultations, euthanasias, lengthy telephone discussions, etc. They are often not aware that veterinary practice is a people-oriented profession.
- **Romanticism.** With some recent exceptions, the wonderful image of veterinary life that has been created by the media does little to prepare prospective students for the actual reality of the job.

Competition is tough and those who are accepted are some of the highest academic achievers in the country. Once started on a veterinary course, we justifiably take pride in becoming members of the relatively small and elite group of veterinary students, and often do not have the time or opportunity for much contact with other university students or disciplines. All through the course the pressure is sustained, involving enormous workloads and high expectations. If we are very keen students, we seldom have time to step back and look at life, or at ourselves for that matter.

When we get into the clinical years, we may be inclined, due to discomfort or self-preservation, to distance ourselves from the emotional side of the work, while still maintaining the veneer of 'good bedside manners'. We are not usually encouraged to discuss or even acknowledge any personal feelings or attitudes about what we are encountering.

Although we often have very good role models in the clinical staff, we are given little formal teaching on being effective communicators or about establishing good human relationships. Since anything left out of the formal curriculum might be regarded as unimportant, it is not surprising that so many of us graduate from Veterinary School not knowing how to communicate effectively with our clients and are entering our profession without the preparation or confidence for successfully managing the emotional (or human) side of our practice.

It is almost predictable then, that a great number of the formal complaints made against veterinary practitioners are not about lack of medical proficiencies, but are actually about a dearth of 'people' skills.

When consultations are limited to 10 minutes per client, as in some very busy practices, it would be difficult for all vets to implement many of the suggestions made in the text. However, when the time is so short, it is important to make every minute quality time. Nurses and receptionists have an essential role in maintaining the continuity of good communication while the vets become involved with the next consultation.

Most vets have had to develop their own approach and standards regarding the management of pet death in practice.

By setting good standards for these crucial aspects of veterinary work, this book will help practitioners develop a methodical and planned approach, thereby engendering a sense of satisfaction at a job well done. This will help to offset the stress associated with most companion animal death.

Companion animals and their owners will also benefit from the thorough and thoughtful approach proposed in this book.

Background information for all veterinary staff

1
Relationships between humans and their companion animals

The diagnosis and treatment of animal health problems is only one side of modern veterinary practice. The primary difference between a good veterinary practitioner and a merely adequate one lies in the former's ability to gauge and understand client-patient relationships. Without this empathic dimension, the veterinarian is not substantially different from a car mechanic or a TV repair man.
(Professor James Serpell, University of Pennsylvania)

Humans are social animals, not naturally adapted to a solitary lifestyle, and are most comfortable being part of a social group. In order to feel fulfilled, happy and safe, most of us have a basic need for interaction with others, and the interactions need not always be with our own species.

BENEFITS OF LIVING WITH COMPANION ANIMALS

Most people who decide to become vets, vet nurses or choose to work in a veterinary practice have probably all benefited in some way by contact with companion animals, and are motivated by a basic fondness for animals and a desire to help them.

That is something the vet staff have in common with most of their clients and is a good starting point for building up an understanding, an empathic viewpoint, of the attachments clients have to their animals. It is not a matter of 'them and us'. Vets, the staff and clients all love their own animals, and have gained from the many ways they have enriched their lives.

Obviously the relationships people have with their animals, and the benefits derived from owning them, depend a lot on the species involved. However, in all cases, there is potential for strong emotional attachment.

Some of the benefits animals may provide that help to improve the quality of our daily life

Friendship
One of the main reasons for keeping an animal is for companionship and many people regard their pets as their 'best' friends. This may pertain to all pet animals, but it is especially the case with species that interact closely with humans (dogs, cats, horses and some talking birds). Even so, there are obvious differences between friendships with a human and with an animal.

- We assume our human friends might be in our lives forever; we know that animals will not be.
- With our human friends, we feel more or less equal; we can debate deep issues.
- We know that we have to behave in a certain way or the human friendship may be threatened.
- Animals are under our control. In the eyes of the law they belong to us (are our 'chattels').
- They cannot discuss things with us, though they do communicate non-verbally.
- They do not demand much from us and they do not usually take offence.
- There is usually a basic comfortable simplicity in the human-animal relationship.

(There are some relationships that are definitely not simple and comfortable, e.g. with over-dependence of some owners on a pet or vice versa when a dog is over-dependent on its owner.)

Emotional support
- The presence of an animal can provide emotional comfort.
- When troubled by circumstances, when we 'fall out' with family or friends, feel moody or depressed, our animals do not get involved in the problems, but seem to 'understand'.
- They appear to love us unconditionally without any expectations that we have to live up to.
- We can be ourselves however we are at the moment, without pretence.

Self-esteem
- By their unconditional and enthusiastic acceptance, animals help us to feel loved and understood, to feel good about ourselves.

- This is particularly important for those with a poor self-image. Approval from an animal may be a start toward self-acceptance and more social confidence.
- Some people enjoy the attention they receive because of their animal; it may be someone admiring their beautiful puppy or it could be about their own image (having a macho Bull Terrier in a chest harness). The image may not be the main reason for keeping an animal, but can be part of the total pleasure of its presence.

Dependable character
- The nature or character of animals is usually individually predictable. This in itself is reassuring in a life full of unpredictability.
- They are often extolled by owners as 'always so gentle, so kind, cheerful, content, boisterous'.
- Some dogs seem to be perpetually happy and this 'good humour' is infectious; people look at them and smile.

Physical safety
- For those who live alone, the presence of an animal can make us feel more secure and less anxious, whether or not that animal could really protect us.
- Big dogs may actually protect us physically and the barking of a dog, whatever its size, may deter burglars.

Touch
- Humans are primates, and use touch for comfort and reassurance, as well as for pleasure and feelings of well-being.
- For some people, circumstances make it difficult to give or receive much touching. Animals can fill this important need.

Relaxation
- Animals can help us to relax. Having an animal stretched out beside us, or curled up on our lap, does seem to make us feel more relaxed.
- Their presence relieves anxiety, and it has been demonstrated that stroking them can lower blood pressure and reduce feelings of stress.

Exercise and activities
- Animals encourage us to keep active. Those who walk dogs will be inclined to take more exercise than they otherwise would.

- There are other ways that animals keep us active, whether it is going to training classes, animal groups or clubs, showing, breeding, or generally playing with and looking after them.

Interaction with others
- Animals are wonderful social facilitators, encouraging us to talk to and be at ease with other people.
- We know that those who walk with a dog are more likely to interact with other people than those who walk alone.

Fun/play
- Whatever our age we still have a child inside and animals help release this 'inner child'. We can fool around without feeling self-conscious and without being regarded as silly.

Nurturing
- Animals help us to fulfil a basic natural urge to nurture.
- By requiring our care and attention, they make us feel needed and useful. Particularly for older people living alone, they might even be a reason for living.
- Some people enjoy the challenge of caring for certain delicate or demanding pets like some exotic birds or reptiles.

Aesthetic pleasure
- Most of us get pleasure from looking at our animals and appreciating their individual attractiveness.
- In the case of some pets, like tropical fish, their extraordinary beauty may be the main reason for keeping them.
- We also derive pleasure from watching the activities of our animals, how they interact with us or with their environment.

Their constant presence
- Animals often represent a constancy in our households. They are family members that do not go off to school, to work or on holiday without us. As long as someone is still at home, the animal is usually there too. First thing in the morning we take the dog out (or let the cat in). If we go out, they watch us leave and celebrate our return with enthusiastic pleasure.
- If we stay at home they are usually aware of where we are, and mostly try and join us in whatever we are doing. In the evening they slump down relaxing with us. Last thing, we attend to their needs and see them to bed, which is very often in our bedroom.

When animals die, people may say, 'the house seems so empty now'.

Being family members

- Children do sometimes refer to their cats or dogs as 'like my brother or sister'.
- Adults may say, 'she/he is our baby'. This often occurs when grown up children have left home and does not necessarily imply a frustrated parent figure.
- Animals somehow extend and complete a family; in fact animals may be the only family a person might have.
- The death of a loved animal is often described as 'like a death in the family'.

Links with nature

- For town and city dwellers, animals provide a link with the natural world and remind us that we are part of nature ourselves.
- They sharpen our awareness of the care necessary to sustain living things.

Education and appreciation

- Animals can help children to value and respect and enjoy the lives of other creatures.
- They can encourage us all to appreciate and enjoy the present time. Although we may be oppressed by regrets about the past and anxieties for the future, our animals appear to live fully in the present; by their sheer enthusiasms, they can usually haul us along, making us share with them the joy of the moment.
- Since their life spans are usually a lot shorter than ours, our animals can teach us about letting go as well as about loving. That is a hard lesson for some.

KEY POINT

There are many different ways animals contribute to our lives, depending of course on the practical limits and limitations of the species involved. An animal does not have to be extraordinary to do all the things mentioned. By being a good dog, cat or other pet, our animals can do these things for us, as long as we take good care of them and treat them properly

SPECIAL ANIMALS

When someone decides to get a pet, they usually base their choice
on two main factors:

- The type of animal they personally prefer and find most attractive.
- How the animal would fit into their present lifestyle.

The actual selection of an animal often depends on availability or
what's on offer, and might be different from what was originally
intended.

Once an animal has been brought home, it is valued as an individual for itself, not just as a cat or a dog (or a rabbit). So every
animal is special in its own way, but some become more special to
their owners than others.

Vets and nurses thinking about their own animals can probably
identify the special ones and may find different reasons for considering each one to be so.

Personal experience is a useful basis for being able to recognize
that some of our patients are extra special to their owners and for
appreciating the particular reasons underlying the owners' strong
attachments.

What makes some animals extra special?

Character/personality
Some animals are just outstanding individuals and even a short
relationship with them can leave a lasting impression. It may be
that they are exceptionally intelligent and responsive. There may be
a mutual understanding, a deep rapport with the owner.

Length of time involved in the relationship
The longer we have an animal, constantly living together, adapting to
each other's ways, the more we become attached. We slip into a long
easy companionship, which may involve a large chunk of our life.

Links with past events or life transitions
A special animal may have been our first animal, a gift on an
important occasion, may have helped us through troubled times,
a bereavement or major trauma. It may have been the one constant
unchanging factor in a life full of disruptions, broken relationships
or changing homes and leaving friends. It may represent our whole

childhood (never remembering home without it) or may be the first shared love object of a young couple.

Links with other people
An animal may represent some sort of link with a person who has died or disappeared from our lives. It may have been owned by them or may represent a shared period or significant event. The death of such an animal may be like the closing of a door, the final break with the absent person.

Shared experiences
When animals are partners in some shared activity, such as in competitions and exhibitions, mountain rescue or police work, they become more and more valued. As the teamwork progresses, important relationships develop. This is particularly the case with the dogs that provide help to people who have problems with sight, hearing or mobility. These assistance animals become very special, acting as close companions, physical helpmates and social facilitators; they maintain a prime role in their owners' lives.

Orphans/rescued animals
We tend to develop very strong bonds with animals we have rescued or raised as orphans. The more of our nurturing and care we invest, the more we become attached and the more they connect with us. These animals often remain special to us throughout their lives, no matter what they are actually like as individuals.

KEY POINTS

- Though every animal is different and special in its own way, some are special over and above others.
- When clients indicate the importance of an animal in their lives, it is helpful to them if you acknowledge that you have heard and understood what they are saying while reassuring them about your interest and care.
- It is important for the vet team to be aware that the illness of any animals, particularly special ones, can cause owners great anxiety and their deaths may often be associated with or result in other significant losses.

Situations where requirement for nursing creates strong bonds

Animals which need particular and extra care
As with orphans, some ill or injured animals need a lot of attention, care and nurturing. Their dependence makes owners feel responsible and they become very involved with the nursing. The more time and energy people invest in the care of their pets, the more attached they become. Obviously, the continuing supportive role of the veterinary team is important for these clients.

Very young animals
Although they may not have had a long time for building relationships, young animals often dominate our lives by their charm, curiosity, innocence and energy. Their demand for constant care and attention heightens our nurturing impulses. When a young one becomes ill, its need and vulnerability is very upsetting for owners. If it should die, the abrupt end to this nurturing may leave owners feeling empty and bereft.

The death may seem so unjust that it may shake people's trust in themselves and in the vets, draining their confidence and making them fearful of a recurrence if they decided to try again. If they do get another youngster, the vet team should be prepared for increased anxiety about things, which might seem to them trivial. It may be helpful if vets can share with clients that they too feel sad when a young animal dies and that they can understand why owners may feel anxious with a new animal.

Injured wild animals
Wild animals that have required a lot of care and attention can become special, and different from all their wild counterparts. It is important to warn clients about getting them too socialized with people, if they are to be returned to the wild. Also warn clients that tamed seagulls and crows, having lost their fear of people, may start 'dive bombing' and frightening children (and even some adults).

Clients with small pets, birds and exotic animals

Relationships with or attachments to other species and exotics may be very strong, and the feelings of their owners just as worthy of attention and concern as would be in the case of dogs and cats. Owners are especially appreciative when their animals, whether hamster, finch or python, are regarded as worthy patients and given good attention, despite their size or financial value.

The relatively long life spans of some of the less common pets (like parrots and tortoises) contribute to strong bonds with their owners.

Birds that speak to and interact with their owners are greatly cherished.

Even vets who are not familiar with the species will make a good impression as long as they express an interest, and show enthusiasm for finding a solution to the animal's problem.

Always keep good reference books in the dispensary, so that you can quickly refresh your memory. Staff should know the expected life spans of their patients.

Be prepared to deal not only with the wide variety of animals that are brought to you, but also with the great variation in the knowledge and expertise of the owners.

Children

- Children who have pets are likely to have animals when they grow up and their attitudes as adults toward the veterinary profession as well as to individual vets are apt to be affected by their early experiences. They will certainly remember the vets who were kind and supportive.
- Children should be treated with the same respect as an adult owner and their experience considered.
- Some are enthusiasts, having extensive knowledge, even breeding and showing their animals, while others may be virtually ignorant of their pets' needs and health care.
- Even when children have obviously neglected or been unaware of some aspects of care, they should be coached in a diplomatic way, without being shamed or made to feel guilty.
- If their animals are seriously ill or die, children should be supported and not blamed.
- This may be their first experience of being responsible for another life and maybe their first encounter with death.
- Children have a tendency to blame themselves when animals (and people) die.
- They may not say much during consultations, may even appear indifferent, but it is important to take time to explain that animals have shorter lives than people and help them understand the cause of death.
- Thank them for caring for their pet and let them know they can get in touch if they have any questions or need to talk. If they are not present, a card is helpful (and appreciated by parents).

- How children are helped at this time may affect their future attitudes not only to animals, but also to death.

There may be a dilemma for vets, since some of these pets are not worth in money terms what the treatment should cost and most children have not the money themselves. Their parents may refuse to pay large vet bills, since it would be cheaper to get another animal. Diplomacy and careful explanations are needed here. Children should not be encouraged to have a casual attitude towards life, nor should they be encouraged to think their parents are cruel and uncaring.

Some practices have a flexible policy on charges in these situations.

Also see Section 4.1.

Specialist clients

- Many people who keep exotic animals or belong to 'fancy' societies are very well informed.
- If you are unfamiliar with a particular species, the owners may even know more than you do about health care, though they will not have your knowledge of pathology and disease.
- If you feel inadequate, be confident enough to say that though you have not had much experience with that species, you will research the condition yourself or make contact with a specialist colleague.
- Do not pretend; the client will know and will lose respect for you.
- Your client will appreciate your honesty and will value your continuing interest.
- Your medical knowledge applies to all conditions, so have confidence in your basic training.
- Show your enthusiasm and interest; co-operate and share your special insights with each other.

Inexperienced clients

- Although most people know something about cats and dogs, many buy other types of pets without knowing anything about their care.
- Vets can make a big difference to the welfare of these animals, by instructing owners about basic requirements for their physical and behavioural needs.
- Have leaflets on pet care available (RSPCA, UFAW, etc.).

- Some practices print regular newsletters, each edition containing information on a certain type of companion animal. These can form a set of information sheets for giving to clients.
- Staff can also be trained to instruct clients on animal care.
- Clients appreciate the enthusiasm and interest, as well as the information.

Owners of dual purpose animals

- Species kept for practical purposes may also interact with their owners, creating strong bonds.
- Horses, ponies, goats and llamas are especially valued in this way.
- Vets should always be aware of the emotional implications if these animals should become seriously ill or die.

KEY POINTS

- Do not let the size or cash value of children's pets affect your attitude.
- Always have reference books (such as the BSAVA *Manual on Exotic Pets*) handy in the dispensary 'just in case'.
- Respect the knowledge of clients with unusual pets; be honest with them, and willing to work together.
- Show an interest and enthusiasm for all types of patient. This is greatly appreciated.
- Be willing to increase your own knowledge and locate local specialist vets for referrals.
- Be aware of clients' emotional attachments to all kinds of animals.

UNSUCCESSFUL HUMAN–COMPANION ANIMAL RELATIONSHIPS

The word 'relationship' or 'bond' may seem to imply a positive or beneficial connection. People usually get animals because they anticipate that some sort of benefit will follow. However, the bond can be broken or never even established, and many animals are discarded or rejected. Because of unsatisfactory human–companion animal relationships, the veterinary profession is regularly involved with the premature death of far too many healthy animals.

The animals lose their lives, the owners are usually very unhappy, often guilt ridden, and the veterinary staff are forced into the emotionally draining and stressful situation of having to terminate healthy lives when all their training has been towards saving and promoting life.

What are the underlying causes of rejection of individual animals?

- The wrong choice of species/breed/individual for the lifestyle or needs of the owners and the purposes expected of the animal.
- Unrealistic expectations for the animal by naïve potential owners who have not considered all the more difficult aspects of bringing an animal into their lives.
- Ignorance about the importance of socialization periods, and behaviour training and resultant behaviour problems are a major cause of dissatisfaction with, and rejection of, animals.
- Ignorance about the needs of the animal, and of the environmental, social and husbandry requirements for fulfilling them. Animals with poor quality of life develop many problems.
- Ignorance about health care. Unhealthy animals are not much pleasure to have around. They may be listless, unattractive and a trouble to care for. Bonded owners usually go to great lengths to nurture and care for their sick pets, whereas a recent arrival in a naïve household may be discarded at the first sign of trouble (e.g. the many Christmas puppies discarded because they developed digestive upsets).

How can vets improve this situation?

- **Advise.** Be prepared to advise potential owners about the choice of suitable pets, the most desirable age, the best place to obtain them and provision of the appropriate care.
- If parents ask for advice, encourage them to get books out of the library, and to join the children in reading about the selection and care of the animals they are thinking about, and making all the arrangements and preparations beforehand.
- **Educate.** When an animal is brought to the surgery for any reason, vaccination or health check, etc., it is an opportunity to help the client in prevention of future problems. Especially for puppies, emphasize the importance of those early (7-14) weeks of socialization, tell the owner about puppy play groups and training classes, and recommend good books and videos on training.

You might even have a small lending library. (See Appendix 3 for further reading.)

- **Review.** Take advantage of the booster vaccinations to find out how the animal is getting on, how training is working and to give advice about any problems before they become entrenched.
- Some practices run their own behaviour clinics or a referral service to a behaviour specialist.
- Involve the practice in community projects, e.g. in connection with local welfare or animal societies. Introduce puppy playgroups for your clients, maybe in co-operation with a local dog trainer. As well as socialising the puppies, these classes encourage bonding and help owners to understand their pets. Talk to schools or local groups about responsible ownership.
- Some practices have more time and commitment than others for these kinds of activities. Those that do involve themselves find that their practice gets the reputation of being caring and responsible.
- Establish connections with individuals and groups involved in training and in animal rescue.

LEARNING ABOUT CLIENTS' RELATIONSHIPS WITH THEIR COMPANION ANIMALS

In order to establish satisfactory connections and maintain good open communications with clients, it is useful to know how they feel about their animals and what role the animals play within the family. This need not take a lot of time, just an increased awareness during routine interactions.

Observation

Observation may give some clues and even reveal quite a lot about the nature of the relationship (it may also be misleading to make anything but tentative assumptions based on a few minutes of attention).

In the waiting room
- The veterinary staff can observe the interaction between the owners and pets.
- When owners are talking to their pets, notice what they say and their tone of voice.
- How does the animal respond?

- Do they caress their pets, making a fuss of them, or are they cool, virtually ignoring them?
- Does the animal seem to be very dependent or more interested in what is going on in the room?

In the examination room
- How does the owner lead, bring the animal in? Do they put them on the table and walk away?
- Do they reassure and fondle them? Do they hold on so tight that it interferes with examinations?

Routine questioning

Do not be in a hurry. Begin by talking about the pet and its problem before getting down to the physical examination.

Even routine questions can provide a great deal of information; just stay with the owner for a moment and maybe follow through with a few more questions.

'How long have you had Smokey?' may give you information that Smokey had been a graduation present 10 years ago or that he had been an abandoned puppy that was still unweaned, etc. If the answer is simply the number of years, you may ask, 'Where did you get him from?'.

You may learn that Smokey had come from a shelter or he may have belonged to a parent who had recently died. When there is an important story connected to an animal, it does not take much encouragement to learn more.

Owners often like to tell about their animals and themselves as well.

Asking, 'who usually looks after Smokey?' gives you a good idea of who else is in the family and what their relationship is to the animal. You may learn that the owner lives alone, or that the wife hates the dog, or that the children, even the 4-year-old, all help to look after it.

Put brief notes on the case sheet. Owners really appreciate that you remember about them.

Comment

Aaron Katcher (a psychiatrist associated with Companion Animal programs at Pennsylvania vet school), when studying clients' relationships with their animals, draws a circle with a dot in the middle. The dot represents the owner who is then asked to place marks representing members of the family, including the pets, in positions near or far away from the centre dot according to how close they feel to them. He believes this tells you a lot about people's attitudes to their animals, as well as being a window into the family dynamics. The animals are often placed closer to the centre dot than other family members!

2

Communicating with clients

Communication is a process of connecting with another person and involves much more than just the words alone. Obviously words are the basis of factual information, but when communicating feelings and thoughts, the tone and inflection of the voice and the visual messages transmitted by body language are more important than the words themselves. It is not only what they say, but how they say it.

WHY IS GOOD COMMUNICATION IMPORTANT FOR A VET PRACTICE?

- Clients may not be able to assess the medical skills of the vets but they do know when they feel that they have been understood, and that both their animals and themselves are valued.
- Good communication results in building a rapport with clients that develops with time and results in bonded clients who consider the vet to be a friend to them and their pets.
- People select and remain loyal to vets with a friendly and compassionate attitude, who care for their animals with kindness as well as competence, and who are good communicators.
- The whole staff have impact on the clients' perceptions about the practice.
- Nurses often do the most communicating, talking with clients before and after consultations, and may have to report difficult news to owners.
- Receptionists, practice managers and nurses are often first in the 'firing line', and have to try and smooth things over when owners have complaints or are angry, especially when the vets themselves are poor communicators.
- Communicating well does not take more time; it saves time, by preventing misunderstandings.

BODY LANGUAGE

- Try to become aware of messages given by body language. Imagine the impact of your own body language on others. (Practise acting out different emotions in front of a mirror to see how it looks and feels.)
- Defensive: crossed arms and legs may be defensive; open arms portray confidence.
- Nervous, anxious: foot or finger tapping, fast blinking, rapid breathing, arms clutching body, tension in voice (maybe high pitched).
- Shocked or stunned: glassy eyed, pallor or flushing, perspiration, difficulty in talking, physical weakness (strong self-control may mask this).
- Depressed: collapsed posture, monotone or dulled speech.
- Embarrassed or unconfident: looking down, halting speech, clasping hands.
- Angry: glaring, sitting back, stopping listening, maybe icy, tight lipped and withdrawn, or flushed, noisy and even violent.

EFFECTIVE COMMUNICATION IN A VET PRACTICE INVOLVES: LISTENING, QUESTIONING AND GIVING INFORMATION

Listening

Is a skill that can be developed and improved by practising self-discipline and self-awareness. Good listening also requires cultivating a capacity for empathy.

Empathy is the ability to understand how the other person feels in his/her world. It is not the ability to assume how you would feel in the other person's situation nor knowledge of how other people have felt in that situation. It is as if you were looking out of the other person's eyes. Of course you never really know what it is like to be them, but if you momentarily step out of your own framework, when you listen to them you can really hear what they are saying.

Basic listening skills involve **attending behaviour**:

- Appear to be relaxed, composed, confident and caring. Assume an open posture.
- Position yourself on eye level with the client. Sitting is better for long or sensitive discussions.

- Remove any physical barriers (like a desk or table) between you and your client.
- Be near enough to establish a rapport or connection with your client. Closing the distance between you makes for more familiarity, but respect the client's personal space.
- Be attentive, making some eye contact, but be careful not to stare.
- Incline towards the client when talking or listening.
- Demonstrate that you are listening by nods, facial expressions and murmurs.

Questioning

Questioning using supportive statements makes listening active rather than passive:

- Questions ('How do you mean? What makes you say that? Could you tell me more?').
- Supportive statements ('I see; Go on, I'm with you; That is interesting, I agree').
- Ask questions to clarify what clients are saying; it tells them that you are really listening.
- Give clients a chance to restate a point that you have not fully understood.

Reflecting means giving back to the client a sense of what they have just said:

- Repeat, in your own words, what you think you have heard (especially about their feelings).
- Be tentative in your interpretation; then you can restate and clarify (for you and them.) This avoids misunderstandings and wrong assumptions.
- Display empathy by using reflecting statements ('You seem upset/annoyed/angry').

Summarizing clarifies and ensures that you have understood ('So what you are saying is? You mean?').
Blocks to listening to clients include:

- Being distracted by external sights and sounds. Be fully confident of the ability of your reception staff to deal with any problems until you have finished consulting.
- Being preoccupied with personal thoughts.
- Worrying about the time (make sure your appointment system allows enough time for a proper consultation).

- Being bored.
- Being distracted by the client's appearance or behaviour.
- Being shocked or disapproving.
- Thinking of the next question, attention not on the present moment.
- Interrupting, not letting the client finish.

Do not:

- Begin your physical examination while the client is still talking to you.
- Turn your back and consult the computer while the client is talking.
- Interrupt or try to finish the client's sentences for them.
- Flick through pages or read notes while a client is talking.
- Look at your watch or clock.
- Eat or drink when you are supposed to be listening.

Questioning to gain information from clients:

- When asking questions, give time for the client to think, and use all your listening skills.
- Ask only one question at a time and wait for an answer before asking the next.
- Ask closed questions (when, where, who) which can be answered with one or two words for factual information or when you are trying to curb long unhelpful explanations.
- Ask open questions (how, what) for eliciting thought and getting more information. 'Are the faeces normal?' may give a simple 'yes'. 'What are the faeces like?' will give you more of a description.
- Follow up verbal clues. You may miss important information by not listening, e.g. the owner of a leukaemic cat may want to tell you that his daughter died of leukaemia.
- Do not be in a hurry to rush to the next question!

Giving information to clients

Be aware that some people need to have a lot of information in connection with any problem situation in life; that is their way of coping. Others cope better with minimal information.

When giving information (information you want to give and that you need the client to comprehend):

- Adjust information according to the understanding and experience of your client.

- Explain simply, in ordinary language, if a client has no medical or biological knowledge.
- Take care not to be patronising; your client may know more than you do about other subjects!
- Use pictures or diagrams or examples to clarify things.
- Give very basic descriptions.
- Use analogies, e.g. in kidney failure compare healthy kidneys to plums, fibrosed kidneys to dried up prunes; the cardiovascular system to the central heating, the heart is a pump, the vessels pipes and the organs represented by the radiators. (People may have difficulty relating to kidney failure and why, due to reserve capacity, current tests do not show up early trouble. Use the analogy of a boat with the water leaking into the bilges under the floorboards, which can only be detected when the level rises above the boards.)
- Repeat and write down important points. Memories are limited, especially with new information. An attending nurse may repeat the main points after the consultation.
- Hand out written sheets or leaflets on specific disease processes or conditions. These may be supplied by commercial firms or produced by the practice.
- Be willing to explain things again to other family members.

The manner in which you deliver information is important:

- This is what makes you different from a computer.
- Speak clearly and slowly. Use a tone of voice appropriate to what you are saying.
- Use appropriate facial expressions, body language. Do not be artificial, just relax.
- Be genuine, honest (congruent in counselling terms). This is crucial to being credible. If you do not believe what you are saying yourself, no-one else will, especially your clients.
- Appear to be confident; if you change your message, explain why.
- Be willing to explain all the risks and costs as well as benefits of what you are offering.
- Be willing to make referrals.
- Avoid terminology that may be misleading, e.g. 'put to sleep' instead of 'helped to die'.

Ask yourself:

- Has the client really understood what I have been saying?
- Would they be able to explain to their family?
- Have all their questions been dealt with?

- Have their anxieties been acknowledged and dealt with?
- Are they feeling confident about my competence?
- Are they feeling that I care about them and their animals?
- Has the client been involved in any decision making?
- Have they been able to make an informed judgement on the information they received?

CONSEQUENCES OF POOR COMMUNICATION

Many complaints against vets are based on poor communication. Common complaints from clients are that:

- They were not given clear explanations and felt confused or uncertain about the diagnosis or the cause of the condition, the choice of treatment, what the treatment was supposed to do, the reason an animal died, etc.
- They had no encouragement or opportunity to take time in considering options; they had not been given encouragement to ask questions and had been rushed into decisions.
- They were not shown respect or consideration.
- The vets and staff did not seem to care.

(Remember that appearing to be aloof or detached is often interpreted as being uncaring.)

SITUATIONS WHERE COMMUNICATION MAY BE DIFFICULT

- Clients with disabilities (see Section 3.2). It may be necessary to adapt your manner of communication according to the abilities of the disabled person.
- Clients from different ethnic backgrounds (see Section 3.3). Sometimes older clients from different ethnic backgrounds are unable to speak or understand English. Usually a younger family member or friend can act as interpreter. Give your attention to the client even though using the other person to translate.

3

Client-oriented practice management

MAKING THE ENVIRONMENT ATTRACTIVE AND WELCOMING

These are ideas that some vets have found useful:

- Make the Reception (waiting area) restful and interesting with plants and attractive paintings of animals and landscapes. These relax people more than educational charts, which can be laminated and bound together with a ring, and taken out when required.
- A beautiful fish tank will be beneficial for stressed clients and educational for staff.
- Have aviaries or tanks with small pets. This reassures owners who have similar pets and is a good way for staff to get familiar with the handling of and caring for these animals.
- Put up a 'rogues gallery' with photographs of patients and cards from owners, or better have some large photograph albums for pictures of pets donated by the clients.
- Some practices have a remembrance corner, with a big album on a table, for pictures of and tributes to loved pets that have died. The staff can put in poems that they think appropriate as well. Clients really appreciate these books and love looking through them.
- Display leaflets about services available (pet loss befrienders, pet fostering services, etc.).
- Have a notice board for general information, services available like puppy classes, behaviour clinics, geriatric screening and for notices of animals needing homes, families wanting animals, missing animals, etc.
- For children keep a selection of attractive soft toys in Reception, letting them choose which one to temporarily care for. These seem to keep the children quieter and better behaved, and are returned after the consultation. Larger toys can be used to demonstrate how to put on 'Haltis' and Elizabethan collars.

- Have some good children's picture books about animals (including a few on pet loss).

If possible, have a small quiet room where clients can have privacy for difficult discussions, for spending some time with a pet before euthanasia or for recovering from an emotional trauma. This room could be used for euthanasia as well. Make it look warm and reassuring rather than clinical. Have a large mat available so that a client can sit on the floor holding their pet during euthanasia.

Ideally, a separate exit allows distressed clients privacy, rather than having to go out through a waiting room full of people. If this is not possible, a room divider may be placed in the waiting room, used both for hanging plants and other displays, and shielding the door to the consulting room, so clients have a bit of cover when leaving the room.

ATTITUDES OF VETS AND STAFF

- The telephone receptionist may be the clients' first contact with the practice and should always sound welcoming and pleasant (if not, that might be the one and only contact).
- All the staff should be warm, friendly and interested in both the clients and animals, giving the impression that everyone cares and that this is a safe place.
- Give clients respect, while being kind, and never be patronising.
- Alert staff to recent deaths or impending euthanasias by posting notices on a small board in the staff room. This will ensure that the owners are treated appropriately when they come in.
- No staff member should be abrupt, moody or insolent, no matter what else is going on in their lives.
- Never talk about the clients when you might be overheard in the waiting room.
- Always try to be aware of the clients' emotional state and act accordingly.
- Be prepared to 'change gear' when a patient comes through the door. Each consultation presents a different story and you need to be flexible, 'selecting a gear' that is appropriate for the situation and for the client's needs. (Going from puppy vaccinations to euthanasias.)
- The vet surgery must always appear to owners to be a safe place for them and their animals.

- If a very distressed owner presents you with an animal, which has obviously been needing and not getting veterinary care, do not be hard on them even though you are angry that an ill animal was not brought in sooner. If they are already upset, reinforcing their guilt will not help.

A vet writes:

> *It seems the experience of many pet owners (particularly older people) that euthanasia is the only solution to a complex problem in an older pet, and that the fear of a possible euthanasia decision may delay the owners from seeking help. It is important to have made your clients confident that you will only suggest euthanasia as a last resort, and only when it is in the pet's best interest.*

GET TO KNOW YOUR CLIENTS

- Your appearance and conduct should convey warmth, confidence and calm control.
- Introduce yourself to the client, act in a manner you are comfortable with and be consistent.
- Clients need to believe they will get the best possible attention, so demonstrate interest, energy and enthusiasm even though you feel harassed or tired.
- By asking basic questions about the animal you can often get a 'window' into the family.
- Address clients in an appropriate way. Some like familiarity and first names; others, especially older people, prefer surnames.
- Introduce the practice to the clients. During quiet periods, offering clients a tour of the practice gives them confidence about entrusting their animals to your care. Hyperactive children can be bribed with the chance of a 'behind the scenes' tour if they behave.
- Encourage clients to bring their children. They are keen to learn and appreciate being able to do things like listen to their dog's heart or look in its ear. While you are explaining to the children what you are doing, the parents are also learning.
- Be prepared for the clients whom you recognize as being exceptionally dependent on their animals or feeling vulnerable for some reason (bereaved, ill, financially compromised).
- Be patient with clients who have had previous experiences and are distrustful of or hostile to vets or staff.

- Be informed about clients who identify with their animal's disorder (cancer, diabetes, etc.).

See also Sections 3.13.3.

Get to know your patients

- Do not approach a shy animal too quickly. Let it explore and get used to being in the room.
- You can learn a lot just watching its behaviour while it is moving around.
- Introduce yourself to the animal in whatever way seems apt (getting down to dog level).
- Call it by its name and always get the sex right (sometimes names are misleading). Try to make your first impression an agreeable one, by making a fuss of it, giving special treats and not poking around or doing anything unpleasant until the animal has relaxed.
- If an animal is frightened of vets, it may help to have a practice uniform that is not white. Sitting down with a client while taking a history seems to give animals more confidence.
- If an animal appears to be unfriendly, make some statement about your understanding that for some, vet surgeries are not the favourite place to be. Do not react with hostility or condemnation.

Dogs

- Approach dogs gently, trying not to intimidate them. Avoid standing or leaning over them.
- Avoid direct eye contact, or staring dogs in the face. Blink when looking at them.
- Stand alongside, facing the same direction as the dogs, rather than in front of them.
- Some dogs, especially big ones, are more comfortable being on the floor than on a table, so do as much as possible down at their level. Talk to owners while crouching by the dogs.
- Soften your face by smiling and laugh with the owners.
- If you feel you have to muzzle the dog, explain that this provides a distraction and takes its mind off the procedure/examination. It is not a judgement on the dog's character.
- When you have learned from experience that a dog is difficult to handle, you can offer the client sedative tablets to be given before the visit.

Cats
- Try to restrain cats with the minimum force and the lightest touch.
- Many cats get frightened because the person holding them is nervous and squeezes them too tightly.
- The more relaxed and confident you can be the easier a cat will be to handle.
- Fondle the cat before doing anything to it. Talk to it and massage its ears, which cats love.
- If necessary, use a special spray that is designed to calm nervous cats

ASPECTS OF PAPER WORK

Case records

Keep up to date information on health insurance cover. Keep updating contact telephone numbers. It is useful to have some extra information on case records (but respect confidentiality).

- Have details of the family, identifying who has immediate care and who is involved with the pet.
- Put in names of family members and even occupations; clients are impressed if you remember things about them. If a spouse leaves or dies, change the title 'Mr and Mrs'.
- Some vets have a code system (**) to alert staff that extra time might be required for a serious situation.
- If an animal is likely to be difficult or dangerous, another warning code may be used. This can be graded: ! = possibly aggressive when stressed; !! = will react aggressively when stressed; !!! = liable to be aggressive without any interventions, take precautions!
- Always record emotionally charged interactions with clients. It is important that both you and your team are able to access the information if necessary at a later date.

Be alert!

When an animal dies, establish routine procedures

One person should have responsibility for checking that all the steps have been properly followed.

- Record the patient as dead on the clinical records.
- Suppress all reminders and recalls.

- Cancel any future appointments that might have been made for the patient.
- Immediately inform all staff and post a notice of the death on the staff notice board.
- Clearly identify the body and establish the client's wishes for the body.
- Determine who will send the condolence card or letter and ensure it is done.

Always do a double check to make sure that the file has been adjusted. Calling a new animal by the dead one's name can be upsetting. Sending vaccination reminders for dead animals is devastating for the owners (and the practice).

Consent forms

Before any procedure requiring admission, sedation or anaesthetic there should be a routine consent form to be signed by the owner. This is an opportunity to explain the risks involved with any anaesthetic, particularly for some species, like rabbits. Some practices recommend a pre-anaesthetic blood test for cats and dogs aged over 5.

Asking clients to sign the consent form before euthanasia takes sensitivity and tact. It is almost impossible to turn such a formal request into a caring moment. It is an area fraught with difficulty and can cause a lot of grief to an unstable client. Some vets feel it is an unnecessary ordeal when the clients are well known, especially if they have had a pre-euthanasia consultation.

In the case of unknown clients who just bring in an animal for euthanasia, it is important to establish ownership as well as getting them to sign a consent form.

Always ensure that clients understand what they are signing for and explain what 'euthanasia' means. If they are upset, it is best if the nurse sits next to them.

Payment
- Paying bills for a loved animal that has died is always distressing and it is especially painful for the owners when the death has been by euthanasia.
- With unknown clients collect payment before euthanasia.
- With well-known clients, be prepared to be flexible. Let them know that they do not have to pay at the time.
- Some clients want to pay and get it over with (they do not want a bill coming in the post as a reminder). They can pay you in the

consulting room, instead of at the reception desk, but this is difficult if paying by credit card.

- If sending an itemised bill, use the phrase 'veterinary services' rather than 'euthanasia' or 'disposal of body'. This may be difficult when information is in the computer program. Write a few personal words to soften the impact of the bill and send it 5–7 days after the death.
- Do not send the bill at the same time as a condolence card, which should be sent within 1–2 days of death.

Information handouts

Giving out information sheets can be beneficial for clients. These save a lot of time and the clients are grateful.

It is impossible for people to remember everything that has been said, especially if they are befuddled from hearing some unpleasant news. Reading about things gives them a better basis for understanding, and thus helps them cope with different situations.

Many practices use their own custom-made information sheets about a variety of subjects (parasite control, neutering, special diets for different conditions, pet identification, caring for different kinds of pets, pet loss, etc.).

Some practices produce a regular newsletter containing information that helps clients care for their animals as well as containing practice news. The practice staff co-operate in collecting material and putting it together. News of staff changes, staff events (like having babies, passing exams, etc.), patients that have won prizes (like pet slimmer of the year), notices of special events, promotions and new services available all help clients to feel part of a practice community. Newsletters are very good public relations and are greatly appreciated by clients.

TELEPHONE COMMUNICATION WITH CLIENTS

The telephone is your most important link with pet owners outside the practice. **Properly managed, it can become your most valuable communication tool.**

General

- Ensure that all staff answer clients' phone calls in a manner that conveys warmth and interest.
- Do not leave a potentially distressing message on an answer phone. Just ask the client to contact the surgery.
- When critical decisions need to be made, it is best not to do this over the phone, but to say something like 'we need your help in making further decisions about Poppy. Will you be able to come in and have a talk?'.

Develop a sound practice telephone policy

- Always have a pen and paper at each telephone in the practice.
- Position a telephone at every computer workstation to ensure that patient and client details can easily be accessed.
- Telephone messages must be properly recorded and conveyed. If possible, try to use your computer system. This will prevent messages getting lost or ignored on loose pieces of paper. If you do not have a computer system, make sure the system you use is reliable.
- Accord telephone callers the same status as someone waiting in Reception – engender the concept of a virtual waiting room. Someone kept waiting at home for you to return a call is as likely to become as impatient as someone waiting for ages in your Reception to be seen by a vet. You can even have a waiting list for this virtual waiting room showing all the people expecting calls or action by members of the veterinary team. It will serve as a constant reminder that they require attention.
- You will need to decide whether it will be your general policy to either contact the client yourself or if you will expect the client to telephone you.

The client phoning you

  Advantages
- The onus is not on you to remember to make the call.
- Saving on outgoing telephone calls?

  Disadvantages
- The incoming call is unlikely to occur at a convenient time.
- Your work can be repeatedly interrupted by incoming calls.
- Staff time is taken up answering the call and locating you to take the call.

- The main practice lines may be jammed by these incoming calls.

If you do prefer to get the client to telephone you, set aside a specific period in your day for taking all incoming calls. Inform your staff of these times and make sure you have no other activities scheduled for this time. Make sure you are situated near a computer workstation so that you are able to look up any relevant details.

You phoning the client

Advantages
- Calls can be made at your own convenience.
- You can properly prepare for the call and have all the relevant details at hand.
- Because you have initiated the contact, you are more in control. This allows you to more easily dictate the length of conversation.
- No other staff time is taken up dealing with these calls.
- You can use telephone lines (such as fax lines and unlisted numbers) to make the outgoing calls, leaving the main practice lines open for other incoming calls.
- Clients are impressed by your taking trouble to contact them.

Disadvantages
- The onus is on you to remember to call them. It often helps to tell them to telephone you if they have not heard from you by a certain time.

Timing
Try to anticipate the time at which your client would most appreciate receiving a call.

- If the client is expecting laboratory results, make sure you contact them as soon as possible after receiving the report. When telling the client when to anticipate results, add a little time to avoid them expecting to hear from you too soon. By adopting this policy of 'under-promising and over delivering', you will be giving yourself the opportunity to attend to the telephone call at your convenience as well as impressing the client.
- If owners have left an animal at the surgery for some procedure or operation, it is good practice to phone them as soon as it is evident that all has gone well, reassuring them and letting them know when they can collect the animal. This saves owners hours of standing by their phones and waiting in anxious suspense.

The call

- Communicate information with sensitivity to the client's needs in relation to what you are saying.
- Being dependent on sounds and words to communicate and exchange information in a supportive or reassuring way means that extra attention needs to be given to the tone of voice and the clarity and speed of your delivery.
- Listen for clues that give an indication of what the client is feeling (angry, upset, relieved) and respond accordingly.
- Long silences may mean the client is too upset to talk, or is just thinking. In this case it may be appropriate to say gently, 'Are you still there?'.

Always remember: telephone callers are often potential clients. Their decision to use you will be affected by the telephone manner of you and the staff.

4

Loss, death and bereavement

Thesaurus: Bereave, deprive (of something that cannot be restored).
When a love tie is severed, a reaction, emotional and behavioural, is set in train, which we call grief.
(Introduction to *Bereavement* by Dr Colin Murray Parkes)

None of us can avoid experiencing losses during our lives. Having an understanding of loss and grief in general terms is helpful as a framework for understanding the feelings and reactions that might accompany companion animal loss. It also helps in preparing us for coping with our own losses, and gives us an insight for helping other people who may depend on us.

LOSS

There are two types of losses that humans encounter in their lifetimes.

'Necessary', development loss

Some losses are a necessary part of development, growth and change. They are natural and necessary, such as being born, weaning, leaving infancy, then leaving childhood and becoming adolescent, growing up, becoming independent, then responsible (marriage, children), retiring, ageing, and maybe becoming dependent again, before dying.

At each 'transitional stage' or time of change, a person is more vulnerable than usual and should other losses occur at the same time, such as a pet death, coping may be more difficult.

Circumstantial loss

These are losses which do not necessarily happen to everyone, though most people will encounter some of these during a lifetime. They are not considered to be a necessary part of development, yet they can eventually become a source of personal growth.

Examples of circumstantial loss include:

- Physical health.
- Mental health.
- A body part, limb or one of our senses.
- Love or a loved person, through death, divorce, other circumstances.
- An unborn child, miscarriage.
- A loved animal.
- A job, income, status.
- A home.
- Reputation, credibility.
- Power.
- Freedom.
- Independence.
- Self-esteem.
- Hope or faith.

The reaction to any of these major losses involves grief. Many losses are inter-related. If someone is permanently disabled through an accident, the losses may eventually include most of those on the list above.

The term 'multiple loss' usually implies a series of losses, not necessarily related, e.g. a woman's marriage is breaking up, she is diagnosed as having cancer, she has a bad car accident, then her dog, which has been her main support in these bad times, dies. This is the last straw and she has a nervous breakdown.

MOURNING AND BEREAVEMENT FOR SIGNIFICANT LOSS

Significant loss usually refers to loss of a close relative or dear friend. Although the following information pertains to human loss, it is also relevant for other serious losses.

Mourning is the process through which a bereaved person copes with loss and is a necessary part of adaptation to loss.

'Grief is the personal experience of loss. (Grief Counselling and Grief Therapy, Worden, 1991)

Mourning following the death is also a social process. Other people may be personally involved in the loss, in support for the bereaved and in rites of passage. There are cultural differences in rituals and traditions, which may affect the outward signs of grief.

Phases and stages or transitions associated with mourning

Key workers in the field of human bereavement include E. Khubler Ross, J. Bowlby, C. Murray Parkes and W. Worden. Although they may describe the process in different ways, they are in agreement about the basic concepts.

Before death: anticipation of death; reaction to news about a terminal condition
Khubler Ross has identified five stages of coming to terms with death which the dying person and relatives may work through. This process begins when hearing about the diagnosis of a terminal condition, but, as each person is different, they have different ways of progressing through their grief.

- **Stage 1:** *Denial, shock and numbness.* The person cannot believe that they themselves or their loved ones are dying. Their denial isolates them. They may think, 'No, this cannot be happening to me!' or 'to us'.
- **Stage 2:** *Anger.* Acknowledging their condition, they may react with anger, 'Why me? Why him/her?'. Anger may be directed at others, e.g. people, doctors or God.
- **Stage 3:** *Bargaining.* Attempting to make a deal with fate to extend their time, maybe until after a special event, e.g. a birth or the return of a loved one.
- **Stage 4:** *Depression.* Preparatory grief and depression. The dying person may withdraw and become less responsive.
- **Stage 5:** *Acceptance.* The client accepts that they are dying, and they and their family prepare for death.

Following death
Reactions of grieving people have been described as involving four phases (Bowlby and Murray Parkes)

- **Phase 1:** *Numbness.* Close to the time of a loss, a period of numbness and unreality helps the mourner to disregard the truth of the loss for a short time. Awareness gradually seeps in rather than hitting all at once.

- **Phase 2:** *Yearning.* There is a pining, grieving and sorrowing, and a yearning for the lost one to return. There may be a tendency to deny the permanence of the loss at some level, although the real knowledge is there too. Anger plays an important part at this time, a protest at the unfairness, at being left, abandoned. There is often some degree of guilt.
- **Phase 3:** *Disorganisation and despair.* The bereaved person finds it difficult to function. Normal activities are altered or suspended.
- **Phase 4:** *Reorganized behaviour.* The bereaved is able to begin putting life back together.

There has been a certain unease with categorising events and feelings in such a definite way, since it creates expectations, which may not be appropriate. There is great variation in the actual process. Each person grieves in a unique way, according to the significance of the loss, the character of the person, the circumstances of the loss itself, other situations and losses in their lives, and the nature of the support available to them.

The progression through bereavement is rather like a roller coaster. It may seem slow, then speeded up, sliding backwards, upside down and generally unpredictable and chaotic at times. It may seem that a person is adapting; then an anniversary or special event will send them spinning again. This is to be expected.

Instead of focusing upon what stages or phases must be endured, Worden prefers to concentrate on the tasks or 'grief work' which are linked with the different stages in the grieving process. This implies more autonomy for the bereaved person; suggesting that there are tasks to be worked through instead of just enduring suffering.

Stage	The grief work or task to be achieved
1. Numbness, shock, disbelief and denial	To accept the reality of the loss
2. Pining and intense grief	To fully experience the pain of grief
3. Recovery	To adjust to an environment in which the deceased is missing
4. Reorganisation	To be able to reinvest emotional energy, 'letting go' of the lost person

Needs

The needs of the bereaved person are:

- For the loss to be acknowledged by self and others.
- To be given permission to grieve, by self and others.
- To be given permission to stop grieving, by self and others.

It is important that vets and all their clinical staff are familiar with the manifestations of anticipatory grief, as well as bereavement following death, in order to be prepared, to understand and to be able to provide appropriate support for clients, whatever their reactions might be.

Reactions to grief

Feelings
- Shock.
- Anxiety.
- Numbness.
- Loneliness.
- Anger.
- Fatigue.
- Guilt.
- Helplessness.
- Sorrow.
- Yearning.
- Fear.
- Sometimes relief.

Physical sensations
- Hollow stomach.
- Muscle weakness.
- Tight chest and throat.
- Pain.
- Over-sensitivity to noise.
- Dry mouth.
- A sense of depersonalisation.
- Lack of energy.
- Breathlessness.
- Lethargy.

Thoughts
- Disbelief that death has happened.
- Preoccupation with thoughts about the deceased.

- Confusion.
- Experiencing the presence of the deceased by seeing them, hearing them, sensing their presence (some people fear they are losing their sanity).
- Difficulty in concentration.
- Self-reproach, assuming responsibility for the circumstances.

Behaviours
- Sleep disturbance.
- Carrying objects.
- Appetite disturbance.
- Searching for and calling out to the deceased.
- Absentmindedness.
- Crying.
- Social withdrawal.
- Sobbing.
- Dreaming of the deceased.
- Revisiting places.
- Avoidance of reminders.
- Restless over-activity, especially cleaning.
- Treasuring objects.

Summary
The following table is an attempt to summarise the needs of a bereaved person following a significant loss, such as death of a partner or child. Since individual patterns vary tremendously, this table is intended only as a guide. These are not true expectations either in the sequence or timings of reactions. General time spans are only suggested; there is no 'normal' time.

 Although this describes bereavement for a loved human, vet staff will recognize many aspects that their clients may manifest (though the intensity and time scale are usually very different).

REACTIONS TO ANIMAL DEATH

Why should vets and staff be knowledgeable about attachments to, loss of and grief for companion animals? As owners ourselves, most veterinary staff eventually experience the death of a loved animal. (So it is not a 'them and us' situation, and it is good to keep remembering that.)

 Most of your clients will sooner or later have to face the loss of their animals and you are likely to be involved. The majority of

Reactions to events	Feelings	What is needed from others	What is needed for self	Possible duration
On learning of terminal illness	Alarm Shock Disbelief Anger	Reassurance Confirmation Friendship Honesty Frankness	Time to adjust and to accept	Hours to weeks
At approaching death	Anxiety Fear Dread Panic Helplessness	To say goodbye Forgiveness? Love	To deal with unfinished business? Forgiveness	Hours to days
On witnessing or hearing of the death	Numbness Shock Relief	Support Protection	Final farewells	Hours to days
(Immediately after death) World may be in chaos	Being lost Helplessness Bewilderment 'If only' Reliving events	Practical support Help Understanding	To face the events; to 'do the right thing' (funerals)	Numbness usually wears off within a month
Early grief Yearning Pining	Physical and mental pain Anguish peaks at 5–14 days Restlessness Searching Anger and guilt	Reassurance Being listened to Acknowl-edgement Talking about/ remembering the dead person	To accept reality of loss To grieve To experience the pain	Days to months
Sorrowing Despair Disorganisation	Anxiety Loneliness Fearfulness Hopelessness Depression Irritability	Patience Tolerance Acceptance Being listened to Allowed to grieve in own way	To let the dead go To forgive and accept self To minimise social withdrawal	This usually persists during first year
'Recovery' Episodic sorrowing	Pangs of grief Gaining energy Nostalgia Sadness	Help and permission to re-establish life Continued contact	To make sense of life without the other To value self To make social renewal	This may take another year
Adaptation Establishment	Coping Acceptance Relief Good memories as well as sad	Normal friendships	To find some purpose in life Fulfilment in new and old relationships	Variable, may take several years

companion animal deaths involve euthanasia. The more understanding you have of your clients' situations and reactions, the
better equipped you will be towards helping them through these
difficult times.

**From the owners' perceptions, how does the experience of losing an
animal compare with the loss of a human?**

Before the animal death

* Knowledge of the shorter life span of animals should prepare
  owners (but usually does not).
* They are more involved in the decision about treatments and the
  options to consider.
* They are often more at ease with their vet than with consultants
  in human medicine, and are more confident about asking
  questions.
* They have to consider the expenses of veterinary care (whereas
  the NHS covers that for humans).
* They have to carry the responsibility for euthanasia decisions,
  some involving healthy animals.

At the time of death

* When the death has been planned, the owner can arrange to be
  there with the animal.

Immediately following animal death

* Some people will be sad or sorrowing for a while, feeling that the
  colour has gone out of life and the house seems empty.
* Others may experience many of the feelings, emotions, thoughts
  and behaviours described in the section on bereavement for
  humans.
* They may even go through the phases or stages associated with
  mourning.

**However, there is usually a great difference in the severity, the
intensity and the time span involved.** The 'whole process' could
involve just days or weeks, though it may take months before
some people are ready to start a new relationship.

While vets and nurses should be prepared for all kinds of reactions, the most usual are:

* **Shock** at the swift transition from life to death.

- **Tears and sobs.** People often say they cried more for the dog than for a mother. This does not imply they loved the animal more, but somehow the fact that it has died is easier to assimilate than the death of a greatly loved human. Sometimes the tears for an animal open floodgates for another deeper grief that is still being worked through. Be aware of this possibility. Acknowledge grief and encourage owners who cry: 'Do not apologize, it is appropriate and a tribute to Zac that that you are weeping for him'.
- **Guilt** is often immediate and powerful and often associated with death by euthanasia.
- **Anger** is not as common a reaction to animal death as it is to human death and is often triggered by poor communication (see Section 6.1).

After death

- Decisions have to be made immediately about the body.
- The clients return to a home that feels empty.

Support from others

There may be very little support from outside immediate family and no tradition of support in the community. It can be a very lonely time. The vet staff may be the only ones who know about the death and loss.

Hurtful attitudes from others

Some people may regard grieving for an animal to be ridiculous, which is very hurtful and damaging. A card or note from the practice acknowledging the loss helps to dispel the feelings of isolation.

'Appropriate' grieving for animals?

It is very difficult to make pronouncements as to what is and is not normal. To many observers, grief for an animal that extends for many months may be regarded as excessive; yet if it were for a human, that time span would be anticipated and accepted as normal.

Whether or not a grief reaction following the loss of an animal is appropriate very much depends on the real significance of that loss. If the animal had been one of the most important relationships in the grieving person's life, then perhaps intense grieving could be regarded as appropriate.

It is important not to immediately classify a grief reaction as abnormal, without first understanding the background to the grieving. Those who cannot understand the possible importance of animals are all too ready to describe such reactions as unnatural.

Complicated grief

Saying grief is 'complicated' often implies that there are added factors or losses which make the death more difficult, e.g. the death of a dog that had belonged to a person's deceased mother, or a dog that had been a shared pet in a marriage that had dissolved.

Ambivalent relationships

Human relationships are complex, rarely ever perfect, especially within families. There may be feelings of irritation, anger, even hate. In human bereavement unexpressed (unacceptable) feelings of anger at the deceased result in guilt at being angry ('one must never speak ill of the dead').

When people develop a loving relationship with an animal, there is not so much ambivalence and repressed anger is not common. Neither do owners usually get angry with their animal for leaving. There is usually an uncomplicated sadness for the ending of an honest and beautiful relationship.

However, human–animal relationships may be less than perfect and ambivalence does occur, with unhappy outcomes. People often lose patience with an animal over some unacceptable behaviour. If this becomes intolerable, or the animal is dangerous, a decision to relinquish, or even destroy the animal may be taken. The resultant guilt often masks any anger that may have been directed at the animal. Instead, the unexpressed anger may be turned inward (doubling the burden of guilt), or occasionally toward veterinary staff. Occasionally this unresolved anger may make it difficult for the person to complete the grieving process.

WHAT MAKES SOME ANIMAL DEATHS SO DIFFICULT?

The section 'Benefits of living with companion animals' (see Section 1.1) mentions things we may miss when we lose an animal which might seem to others to be an ordinary, unremarkable animal. In other words, we miss the 'dogness' of a dog, the presence of a dog in our lives and we adapt to that loss in our own way. But of course we miss much more; we miss that special individual animal, and all the connotations it has had for us.

There are three main factors which influence the reaction people experience when losing a pet. Each one contributes to the difficulty and when it is two or all three together, the vet team should be prepared for a delicate situation that requires time and understanding.

- The **'specialness'** of that animal – the importance that specific animal has held for the person involved and the closeness of the attachment or bond between them.
- The **human factors** – the age, stage in life, circumstances and vulnerability of the individual, including life experiences, and personal coping mechanisms.
- **Circumstances of death or loss.**

The 'specialness' of the animal

See 'Special animals' (Section 1.1).

Human factors

Age and stage in life of the person involved

If we recall early memories of our first pets and then follow through our relationships with our animals over our lifetime, we notice that at different times, the emphasis on what we most valued might be different. (Children may delight in having something of their own to care for, whereas a busy parent of five may not particularly relish that aspect.)

- Children often say their animal is their best playmate, or even like a sister or brother. Teenagers may feel that their animal is the only one in the world who understands them (see Section 4.1).
- For young people, in the turmoil and stress of finding jobs and partners, the predictable easy relationship with an animal may be an important steadying influence.

- People living alone at any age rely on their animals for company and companionship. This has increasing significance as people get older and their participation in work or leisure may become limited, and relationships with others decline.
- For very elderly people, who have outlived friends and partners, their only significant relationship may be with an animal.

Life circumstances and individual vulnerability
Life inevitably involves losses and difficult transitions. Some people are better at coping with loss than others. The cheerful presence of a loved animal often supports people through the difficult times. If the death of an animal coincides with or follows other traumatic events, it may seem like the 'last straw'.

People who may be particularly vulnerable at the time of losing an animal include:

- Those recently bereaved or those who have not 'worked through' previous losses.
- Those going through difficult times (exams, fractured relation-ships, etc.).
- Those living lonely lives, without much support from others.
- Those who experience difficulty in relating to other humans.
- People isolated by health problems, especially chronic illnesses.
- People with mental health problems, whose animals may be the only ones who are able to give them unconditional approval and love, and act normally towards them.
- People with physical incapacities, especially those whose animals have helped them to lead more independent fulfilled lives (see Section 3.2).

Circumstances of death or loss

Whether the death is of a human or an animal, the cause and circumstances of a death have an impact on the immediate reaction and the grieving process that follows.

Sudden unexpected death
An unexpected death especially of a healthy individual is always difficult to accept. The period of shocked disbelief, of not being able to absorb the reality of the situation, is always more pronounced when death is unexpected.

Anaesthetic death of apparently healthy animals undergoing
optional or routine procedures
Recommend a pre-anaesthetic blood test for animals over 5 years.

- This is a most devastating situation for everyone concerned. It can certainly shatter the confidence of young, inexperienced vets, and senior vets should be very understanding and supportive.
- This does happen and it is vital to pre-warn owners about the risks of anaesthetics. This is done routinely when the owners sign the consent form for a procedure. This does not help the owners to cope with the death, but it is negligent not to have cautioned them. Rabbits are particularly vulnerable.
- The owner should, if possible, be contacted immediately, not left to find out when coming to collect the animal.
- Breaking the news should be done by the vet involved, or the vet in charge of the practice.
- Be prepared for shock and disbelief, then floods of questions when the news has sunk in.
- It is better to discuss things with the owner in person, rather than on the phone.
- Let the owner know how sad you feel, but do not assume blame. If they just cannot accept it, say that these deaths happen in human medicine as well, such as parents losing children and never understanding why.
- Do not make any charges. Depending on the client, some vets offer to pay for a private cremation when that seems appropriate. Some clients may interpret this as a sign of guilt.
- Be aware that the staff feel sad, even guilty, as well, and encourage everyone to talk it out.
- Help others with what to say if clients keep phoning back, which they tend to do.

Acute medical conditions
Conditions like torsion of the stomach or Parvo infection in pups may be fatal after a few hours and are hard for owners to accept. They may feel that the vets were at fault, and need time and gentle discussion to be persuaded that everything possible had been done.

Violent deaths
Many cats and dogs die on the roads or in some other violent accidents. They may even be shot or possibly killed by another animal. The bodies may be horribly mutilated and, if seen, remembered with lasting horror. If you are involved, try to cover the mutilations with a blanket and especially protect any children

from seeing things which will haunt them later. If appropriate, reassure owners that the animal probably was not aware of what was happening, and death was quick.

Guilt compounds the grief over a sudden death

Many owners feel directly or indirectly responsible for the death. A door left open, a loose collar, a lack of observation, etc. They are often left with many questions 'What could we have done wrong?', 'How could this happen?'. For an owner, a lifetime of responsibility for an animal's care and welfare includes the end of its life as well, and this often leads to a great anxiety and guilt.

Veterinary involvement and attitudes

When veterinary surgeons and staff are involved in the death of animals, especially during euthanasias, their actions towards the animals and owners have important immediate implications. Euthanasias are always difficult for owners. When they have been handled skilfully, with both animal and owner treated compassionately, euthanasias can be thought of as generous acts. Though the owners grieve the loss, there may be very little guilt or anger.

A vet writes:

> *I agree wholeheartedly with the observation that we receive more thanks for killing pets than for curing them. I have probably received five letters after a euthanasia for every one I get for successfully treating a case.*

Difficult euthanasias

When euthanasias have been handled clumsily or things have gone wrong, especially if distressed animals are struggling as they die, owners may have great difficulty in coming to terms with the death. Owners who witness their sick or injured animals dying in apparently great pain or misery, retain the image of those last few minutes for years. This may contribute to a continuation of grieving and an inability to be at peace.

Euthanasia of healthy animals demanded by law

When a loved pet has got among sheep, or bitten someone, it is very likely that they will face a death sentence, which a vet will have to carry out. The Dangerous Dogs Act has been responsible for the unnecessary deaths of animals that never did bite anyone but just happened to resemble a certain breed. This is incredibly tough on owners, who are shocked, sad, guilty and sometimes angry, all at once. The vet staff involved should be aware of just how hard these situations are and should be understanding.

Animals that have disappeared
These are losses with no opportunity for closure; anxiety and worrying compound the grief (see Section 4.3).

Issues related to euthanasia and animal death

1

Reasons for contemplating euthanasia; options to consider

EUTHANASIA OF HEALTHY ANIMALS

There are ethical, emotional and welfare issues for everyone to consider.

- When healthy animals are presented for euthanasia, ethical considerations need to be acknowledged with regard to the animals, the owners and families, the vet staff, and the wider community.
- Vets being advocates of the animals have a responsibility to consider each situation carefully, suggesting other options where possible.
- Killing healthy animals may lead to moral stress and burn-out, especially in those vets working in animal shelters.
- Practices that make an effort to save lives gain respect from and show a good example to the local community. Some practices have a 'no kill' policy for those animals which could be good pets, given the right circumstances.

Unwanted animals

Many healthy normal pets are brought in for euthanasia for a variety of circumstantial reasons, rather than any major problems or deficiencies of the animals themselves.

Find out
Why is the animal no longer wanted?

- Impulse buying. 'Easy come, easy go'.
- Unrealistic expectations about pet ownership, lack of previous experience.
- Unwanted gifts.
- Trivial excuses such as shedding hair, muddy feet on new carpet.
- Family disputes. A dominant family member may decide to get rid of an animal, but others may be unhappy about that decision.

- Family traumas, separation. Often people whose lives seem out of control, cannot cope with and will discard an animal.

What is the relationship of animal with family?

- Who has been the main care giver?
- How do the rest of the family feel? Are there children involved?

Action
- Assess the situation.
- Educate clients. It is best not to alienate them initially by condemning their attitudes. Try to understand their viewpoint, and then work with that to suggest possible strategies. 'I can see how you are feeling, but let us see if we can give this animal a chance.'
- If they have children, warn them of the possible consequences of killing their child's 'friend'.
- Educate clients about how to have a better relationship with an animal.
- You may persuade them to persevere (in cases where is a good outlook).
- If the animal has a good temperament and is healthy, suggest options for rehoming.
- Keep an up to date list on the notice board of clients looking for animals and animals looking for homes.
- Provide a list of local animal rescues and shelters, or pure breed rescue societies.
- If you say that you are going to euthanase an animal, then you must do so.

Young unwanted puppies and kittens
If these are weaned and healthy, most practices will refuse euthanasia. Supply owners with the name of local animal rescue shelters which will usually find suitable homes for healthy youngsters.

Unweaned animals require care, time and dedication. Some practices have connections with volunteers who will help raise and find homes for orphans and abandoned youngsters.

Comment
Vet practices have differing policies about euthanasia of healthy animals. Some have a 'no kill' rule unless an animal is ill or dangerous ('I did not study for 5 years to become a murderer!'). Others feel that it is a vet's responsibility to carry out owners' wishes and that an easy death is a better alternative to the owner dumping it or the possibility of a bad rehoming. It is useful to establish a practice

policy to enable informed action, while still being prepared to assess each individual situation. It is important that practice policy is accepted by all the staff, otherwise there can be frequent conflicts. This should be a factor to consider when joining a practice.

Changed circumstances in owners' lives

- **A change of job or accommodation** may not fit in with keeping animals. Lifestyle may change (moving, travelling, leaving the country).
- **Elderly or disabled people may go into sheltered housing** or other dwellings with 'no pet' rulings. Enforced separation from their loved animal companion can be devastating. They are faced with the choices of killing or rehoming their animal, or continuing to live in accommodation which is no longer satisfactory or safe for themselves.

Find out

Decisions should not be taken without first approaching the authorities involved to see if the situation might be negotiated. In some places new animals are not allowed, but existing ones can accompany their owners. Possibly an alternative residence could be found where the rules are more compassionate. (The Anchor Trust Sheltered Housing Group have information on accommodation that will accept pets. They state that 71% of vets and animal sanctuaries surveyed agreed that older people often have to get rid of their pets needlessly before moving into a residential home).

If housing cannot be found, then maybe a good home can be found for the pet. Owners often worry that their old pets will not adapt to new people. However, some animals adapt remarkably well and make good companions for other seniors.

Often adoptees keep in touch with the previous owners. This lessens their worry but does not reduce the longing for their pet.

Action

- Some vet practices will make a direct approach to the housing management or association, or to the manager of a nursing home.
- Contact the Anchor Trust for advice.
- Help to arrange adoption, through practice and client network, notice board, etc.

Illness of owner

When people live alone (with their animals) and become ill, perhaps needing hospitalisation, there may be no one to look after their animals. These situations cause stress for the owners and may have implications for their health. Although some animals might be taken to a shelter, some are brought in for euthanasia.

Clients who are HIV-positive or who have AIDS may be in a quandary about keeping their pets, bombarded by conflicting opinions and advice from family, friends and health professionals. It is especially important that, at a time when many of their human contacts may become estranged, their animals remain with them to provide unconditional companionship.

Vets can give these clients expert guidance on how to ensure that they minimise any risk of contracting a zoonotic disease from their pets. They should be advised to be particularly rigorous about flea control and keeping vaccinations up to date. Like any other owner who becomes ill, they will need to arrange for help with exercising, grooming and feeding their pet – not forgetting someone to collect pet food or have it delivered. If the prognosis for the client is terminal, they should be supported in making practical arrangements for the future care of their pet.

Find out
● Who is legally in charge of the animal?
● What alternatives have already been explored?
● Is the animal in reasonable health?

Action
Advise carers about Pet Fostering Services which are becoming more widely available or of other charities which have an agreement with the social services to provide kennelling.

Encourage carers to reassure people that their animals can be well looked after and they will be kept informed (and do so).

Death of an owner

Families in grief may react on impulse and demand euthanasia, not being able to cope themselves with the burden of an extra responsibility, or thinking that the animal cannot adapt. They may transfer their own feelings of despair onto the animals and think they would be better off dead.

Find out
- Details about the family and the situation with the animal.

Action
- Encourage the family to take some time with this decision, even arranging some alternative accommodation while they are trying to come to terms with the death.
- Warn them that a hasty decision about a loved one's animal may lead to remorse later. Sometimes other family members or friends will decide to adopt the animal.
- Reassure them that most animals adapt very well to new circumstances, and their last gift to the deceased may be to ensure a good home for their animal.

Comment
If someone who has been recently bereaved, and appears to be overcome with grief, brings in an animal to be euthanased, this might be an impulsive preparation for their own suicide. Being responsible for the care of their animal may just be the one thing that is keeping them alive. Try to use some delaying strategy.

A vet writes:

> *On several occasions I've had owners make requests regarding their pets in the event of their own death. Some have asked me to see that they are taken care of, others have asked me to euthanase the pets. This may have legal implications if it is included in the will.*

In these situations the family might want to have a say in the matter. The lawyer should be consulted. There may be some flexibility and the animal may not have to be euthanased.

Allergies in the family

This is a complex issue. Some physicians advise getting rid of pets without actually being sure the health problem is directly related.

A vet writes:

> *I put down two Siamese cats in response to a doctor's diagnosis of allergy to cats. I found out later that the absence of the cats made no difference whatsoever to the child's allergy! At the time I did not think of suggesting that the cats be placed in a cattery for a trial period.*

Find out
- Would the family really like to keep the animal?
- How serious is the allergic response?

Action
Inform them of other measures to keep down allergens.

- Keep the animal out of bedrooms.
- Groom regularly outside (by a non-allergic person).
- Remove all hairs and dander from carpets and furniture.
- Replace, if possible, carpets with wooden or tiled flooring.
- Reduce general allergen sources in the environment, e.g. dust mites, mould.
- Suggest they might try alternative kennelling for a month and see if the symptoms of the 'allergy' continue.

If the allergy is severe, suggest options for rehoming. Killing the animal may lead to family traumas and a burden of guilt on the allergic person.

Ignorance about disease, health worries

A worried mother may bring in an animal for destruction because she has heard that children may 'go blind from dog worms'. This happened a decade or so ago when anti-dog scare stories were common in the press. It could happen again. Reassure owners, educating them about hygiene and disease control for their pets.

Behavioural problems: a frequent reason for euthanasias

Clients whose pets behaved badly used to be viewed by many veterinary surgeons as time-consuming eccentrics, best referred to a local dog trainer, or they dispensed stock remedies like ACP and castration. Nowadays, behaviour is seen as a window to the overall health of an animal and of its relationship with the family.

My experience is that behavioural cases justify the same levels of effort and enquiry as any other sphere of veterinary medicine because many moods and reactions of animals are directly or indirectly related to disease processes. Thorough clinical examination may reveal previously unsuspected sources of pain, neurological and endocrine disorders, dietary hypersensitivity, sensory impairment or even poisoning.

The veterinary surgeon who conscientiously turns every therapeutic stone assumes the role of ally to the animal, and helps an owner reluctantly accept the euthanasia option if this has to be. The sense of failure and sometimes anger that so often prevails when a young, otherwise healthy animal is euthanased need not worsen the grief of those who have had to lose their pet because of its behaviour.

(Dr Roger Mugford, The Animal Behaviour Centre)

More young dogs die from euthanasia for behaviour problems than from any other single cause.

Animals may be destructive, socially unacceptable or dangerous. Even though they cause great problems, some owners are often strongly bonded and are willing to put up with a lot of disruption before seeking euthanasia.

With the exception of dangerous dogs, pets with behaviour problems should only be declared beyond redemption by someone qualified to make that judgement.

Many problem behaviours involve a clinical condition, which once recognized, could be cured.

Find out
- The history of the problem and the consequences for the family.
- If the animal is potentially dangerous.
- If the owners have already made attempts to modify the behaviour.
- Have the owners consulted a behaviour specialist? What was his/her opinion?
- Are the owners willing, even keen to look at options other than euthanasia?

Action
- Make a thorough examination of the animal to rule out any clinical causes for the behaviour.
- Advise training or behavioural modification in cases where it seems indicated, such as destructive, over anxious or excitable animals.
- Give details of reputable local specialists dealing with problem behaviours.
- Warn owners that some who set themselves up as behaviour experts may not be reliable.
- Inform owners that animals with behaviour problems should only be rehomed where the adopting family understands the situation and is willing to work with it.
- Explain that when an animal is dangerous, euthanasia is really the only responsible option.

- Be aware that the decision to have their animal put to death is very difficult for families who have loved them, in spite of everything. Try to help resolve their guilt before euthanasia takes place.

Preventing these situations
You might:

- Develop your own knowledge about behaviour. Attend workshops, join groups.
- Educate clients about puppy training and socialisation.
- Introduce behaviour therapy into your practice services. Many animals and owners can be helped before the situation gets so fraught that euthanasia is considered.

Animals which do not fulfil the task required of them

For example, sheep dogs or gun dogs that do not work well. Some young dogs could be good pets, others may not adapt. These owners are usually pragmatic and not emotionally committed.

Find out
The dog's age, behaviour, character and previous experience.

Action
If appropriate, suggest options, as above. (The practice may need to make the arrangements, as these owners probably will not.)

Comment
Some practices are well geared up with local connections to find good homes for an occasional animal. Many practices have a flexible policy on these. Some animals, however, such as racing greyhounds, are a problem. If they have been kennel raised, they may not be suitable for house pets, although there are exceptions.

Beware of certain animal lovers who cannot resist collecting many unwanted pets. They often cannot care for or feed them properly and it becomes a welfare issue.

Death imposed by law

Dogs that have attacked people may have been provoked and may have no past record of any aggressive behaviour. Some very gentle, sweet dogs may attack and kill sheep. In both cases a death sentence for the dog may be the result.

Owners may be in a state of shock and disbelief, as well as grief and guilt. They not only lose their dogs, but have to carry the guilt and the consequences for the damage. They may be regarded as being irresponsible even though it was a mischance.

Dogs condemned under the Dangerous Dogs Act may be seized or under orders for destruction. There is a great deal of frustration, anger and guilt associated with these cases.

Find out
The specific circumstances involved.

Action
- Empathise with the owners and families of these animals. The last thing they need is a cold reception or a lecture on responsible pet ownership.
- Acknowledge the difficulties and trauma they must be having.
- Perform euthanasia with great sensitivity, speaking to the animal kindly.

Case report
A 75-year-old man who had recently lost his wife had a friendly 10-year-old Doberman. The dog was tied to the garden gate while his owner went inside for something. A boy came up, teasing and taunting the dog, which bit his finger. Just after the police served a warrant on the man to have his dog destroyed, the man had a heart attack and died.

EUTHANASIA TO END THE SUFFERING OF SICK, INJURED OR DEBILITATED ANIMALS

Apart from severe emergency situations, euthanasia should only be considered after careful assessment of all the relevant facts, taking into consideration the animal's distress and the prognosis based on clinical signs.

The finality of euthanasia can make it a tempting resolution to a difficult medical or surgical case. Always ask yourself if a second opinion or referral to a specialist might not save the patient's life.

How much suffering should an animal endure, before euthanasia is proposed? It is not always simple.

The needs of the owner sometimes are in conflict with those of the animal.

As advocates of animals, vets have a role in educating clients about their animals' welfare in a caring manner that helps clients to make wise, and humane decisions.

Albeit the final decisions are the owners' prerogative, vet opinions, if offered skilfully and compassionately will usually be accepted.

Sick animal presented by a new client

A new client to the practice asks you to euthanase a sick animal. An owner may have heard that you do home-based euthanasia or their own vet may be unavailable.

Find out

Who is the official owner of the pet, what has been the history of the illness, what has led to a euthanasia decision and is that what the owner really wants.

Action

- Contact the previous vet to discuss the case.
- Make your own examination of the animal and diagnosis of the condition, before taking on the responsibility of the animal's death.

Comment

Important personal and professional ethics are involved here and the situation may be quite tricky, involving great diplomacy if you have considered the decision for death to be premature.

Diagnosis of inoperable or untreatable conditions

Unprepared owners need time to adjust to information.

Find out

What the owners think about the condition and about the animal's well-being. It helps them to talk about it and in a way prepares them for your comments.

Action

- Avoid using emotive words when first introducing the idea of there being a serious problem. (Instead of cancer, say a lump, a swelling, a growth.)

- Encourage them not to make decisions when in a state of confusion.
- Provide time for asking questions, exploring all options.
- Involve the family in the discussion.
- Time spent on issues before death prevents guilt and 'if only' thoughts afterwards.

Comment

It is useful to have information to assist in the decision making. Taking a blood sample is seldom a big inconvenience to the pet, yet can yield an enormous amount of objective and measurable data. It often helps to have some numbers to show just how serious a case is. 'Mrs Smith, we've tested Bertie's kidneys and found his creatinine levels are seven times the normal upper limit. This suggests there is little we can do to help him.'

Treatment questionable for welfare of animal

Where treatment might prolong life, but would involve invasive measures which could be questionable for the welfare of the animal.

Prolonged treatment or invasive surgery may buy extra time for an animal, but at what cost (to the animal and the owners) and what are the future prospects for a good quality of life?

Find out

What do the owners really want? Though the outlook is poor, some owners may feel guilty if they do not try everything. It may clarify issues to question for whose benefit would the treatment be? For the animal itself? For the owner or for neither?

Action

Let the owners know that you understand their difficulty and warn them of the probability that there will be some guilt with whatever they have decided to do. Encourage the owners to empathise with the animal, stressing quality of life and poor prospects.

Terminally ill animals not responding to therapy

When animals which have been undergoing treatment are no longer responding and their condition is gradually deteriorating.

Owners who have been determined to do everything possible for their animal, having made a great emotional and financial investment in their therapy, often have difficulty in accepting that there is no longer any possibility of recovery.

Animals often seem very poorly, but then may rally a bit, giving the owners some small touch of hope. As those good moments get less, and the distress or withdrawal increases, then the course of action becomes clearer.

From the time of the initial diagnosis (as in cancer) through the course of treatment, owners may experience the 'anticipatory stages' of grief (shock, denial, anger and despair, and finally resignation, even acceptance).

The more an animal is considered to be the owners' 'baby' (the more personhood attributed to it), the more difficulty the owners might have about letting go.

Find out
Prepare yourself by reviewing the stages of anticipatory grief.

Action
• Scheduling of euthanasia is usually a joint decision between owners and vets. Vets decide from the clinical evidence, and owners from an understanding of their animals and an intuition of knowing 'when the time has come'.
• Give the owner permission to let go which is difficult when the condition has involved gradual deterioration.
• The vet who has cared for the animal and helped the owner through the illness, now has a responsibility to support the owner through the euthanasia as well.

Comment
Sometimes owners are reluctant to let go. If you are anxious about the welfare aspects of keeping an animal alive, another opinion often helps (possibly by asking a colleague in the practice to examine the animal and express their own concern as well).

When treatment is indicated, but it is too expensive for owners and no insurance is available

An animal has a serious condition which could be treated successfully but the clients are unable to pay. There should be a practice policy. Vets are in the business of saving lives and there should be some way to work around a situation.

Find out
If there is a PDSA, Blue Cross or other charity clinic available. If so, are the owners eligible for their services?

Action
• Suggest options (Blue Cross, PDSA).
• Owners may organize a 'whip round' from friends and relatives.
• The practice may allow the bill to be paid in instalments or by bank standing order.
• In some areas, RSPCA, NCDL or Tail Waggers Trust may be approached to help.

Comment
With technical advances, more sophisticated procedures help in diagnoses and treatment, and may prolong life, but inevitably involve more expense, which may be prohibitive for some clients. (Possibly expenses could be kept down by using low tech methods.)
    Knowing that treatment could be a possibility but it is out of reach makes it all the more difficult to come to terms with an acceptance of euthanasia. Prolonged guilt, self-recrimination, and family disputes often follow. In cases where the outlook would be questionable whatever the treatment, the families should be reassured that euthanasia was the kindest option. This helps relieve guilt.

When owners are unwilling to pay, although the outlook for the animal could be satisfactory

Find out
• Is the person with the animal the primary caregiver?
• Have all the family, especially any children, been consulted and considered?

Action
Careful discussion and encouragement to empathise with the animal, may help owners to change their minds about treatment. (They could be offered the suggestions made above.)

Deteriorating quality of life, through ageing, progressively debilitating conditions

There are many issues to be considered, the foremost being the demeanour of the animal itself. Some animals, which are not actually suffering, can adapt to a fairly restricted lifestyle and seem content as long as they can be around their owners.

Find out
- How is the animal's quality of life?
- How are its sensory faculties?
- Has it lost muscular control of bowels and bladder? (Not only difficult for owners, but can be troubling for previously clean animals.)
- Are elderly animals suffering mentally, while still appearing to be fairly healthy? Have they become disorientated and anxious, sometimes barking incessantly when left alone, unsettled, restless, whining and crying?

Action
- Be prepared to spend time with owners in discussing options and decisions. Just as in Alzheimer's, it is very distressing for a family to witness changed behaviour in their animals. If animals are mentally deranged, but still eating and physically intact, their desperate owners who just cannot cope, feel guilty about considering euthanasia and need help with decisions.
- Encourage owners to look from the animal's viewpoint – is it really enjoying life at all? List all the things that are causing the animal difficulty and suffering, both physically and mentally, and then the things that still give the animal some pleasure. This may help in deciding the right time.
- Make suggestions for owners who want to persevere: Flexileads for walking deaf, blind dogs, mobility carts for posterior weakness, nappies for incontinence.
- If euthanasia is planned, warn owners that some old, blind, deaf and confused animals may be frightened when restrained.
- Explain that they may be disorientated like senile people, but are not in pain.
- Some conscientious owners have great difficulty with decisions which appear to put their own interest before that of their animals. They often go to extremes in self-deprivation in order to do the right thing.
- At times, their own welfare and stability is threatened, which also has a negative effect on their animals.

Owners such as these often need to 'have permission' to consider their own needs, and to be reminded that their own unhappiness may result in distress and anxiety for the animals, who love them above all else.

Comment
A vet writes:

> *I find owners are often confused between pain and suffering; they often lump the two together. Suffering can be emotional as well as physical. I am always keen for them to appreciate that suffering does not have to involve pain as such. A patient with severe kidney failure will be feeling awful but will not necessarily be feeling any pain. Similarly, a patient with severe lung problems will be feeling as if each breath is the last but may not be in any pain at all. Relief from pain is not the only justifiable reason for euthanasia.*

Case study – permission needed
A woman phoned the help line in order to talk through a distressing situation involving her Alsatian dog. He had a progressive paralysis of the hindquarters, and had lost bladder control and the ability to walk. Though she was not strong, the owner was assisting him as he struggled outside to defecate. He whined and became restless if she left him, so she was sleeping beside him on the living-room floor. She was continually cleaning him and his bedding so that he did not get sores.

Because the vet had reassured her that the dog did not seem to be in pain, she felt that she could not consider euthanasia and just had to carry on with this caring. She was tired, exhausted and felt on the verge of collapse. The befriender observed that neither the dog nor herself seemed to be having any quality of life and that pain was not the only indication for euthanasia. She suggested that the owner talk it over with the vet. Two days later the woman phoned and said that the vet had been really kind and had euthanased the dog. She was feeling sad but content that the right thing had been done. Her observation was 'I needed permission to think about my own welfare as well as my dog's'.

For those who want their animals to die naturally

It is important to spell out just what that might involve in their particular case. With some conditions an animal could have a very tough passage with organ failure or build up of toxicity.

Just because they are at home does not mean that the family will be there at the death. Unless owners stay with them constantly, even sleeping with them, animals at home are more likely to die alone, whereas with planned euthanasias the owners can arrange to be with them.

Severe injury; emergency euthanasia

Owners are usually shocked, stunned and may be temporarily incapable of rational thought.

Find out
- Are the people who brought the animal the actual owners?
- Is the actual extent of the injury immediately life threatening?

When animals have been badly injured (e.g. a fractured spine, crushed skull) a quick painless death may be indicated and the owners helped to accept the necessity of immediate euthanasia. Some injuries can appear so gross, that horrified owners may demand euthanasia before actually considering options. This is especially so when the indications would be for amputation of a limb or tail, or enucleation.

Action
- Remain calm, caring and confident, containing the owners' alarm. After assessing the situation, give information about possible options. Allow time for them to process information, speaking slowly and repeating important aspects.
- Acknowledge their distress, and answer questions calmly.
- When amputation or enucleation is the issue, reassure them about immediate pain control and the long-term outlook. Stress the adaptability of animals and the ultimate acceptability of their appearance. It helps owners to see photographs of patients that have undergone such surgeries or to be put in touch with the families of these patients.

Comment
In one vet practice whose policy is not to euthanase potentially viable animals (such as those requiring only a tail, single limb amputation or enucleation), they find most owners 'come around' to accepting surgery. Sometimes these animals are kept hospitalized until their appearance is more acceptable and their stitches have been removed.

2

Breaking bad news

Bad news is always going to be bad, but the way you reveal it may make a big difference to the way your client can adjust to it. Imparting bad news is a skill requiring empathy, caring and confidence.

WHY IS IT SO DIFFICULT FOR VETS (AND NURSES) TO TELL PEOPLE BAD NEWS?

- Fear of being blamed by others and of blaming oneself.
- Fear of not having all the answers (especially true of recent graduates).
- Discomfort in dealing with emotions, both personal and of the clients.
- Insecurity due to lack of specific training and experience.
- Fear of saying the wrong thing (e.g. 'I'm sorry' could be interpreted as an admission of guilt, rather than an expression of sympathy).

WHAT HELPS?

- The knowledge that you have done your best, that success cannot be guaranteed and there are limits to what can be achieved.
- Knowing that the bearers of bad news are often blamed; not taking it personally.
- Gradual acceptance that emotions are normal and have a purpose.
- Becoming comfortable with your own emotions.
- Being able to acknowledge emotions in a controlled way.

WHEN THE OWNER IS TOTALLY UNPREPARED FOR BAD NEWS

Sick animals

An animal is presented in an advanced stage of terminal illness or maybe has a condition which appears to be inoperable or un-treatable. Use great care; examinations should not be rushed, nor diagnosis pronounced abruptly.

Find out

While taking a full history, establish who is the primary care giver and who else is emotionally involved with the animal. Check previous records for details of any health insurance.

Action

- After making a preliminary examination, warn the owner that you are concerned about the animal's condition. Lead into the possibilities gently, showing that you care by your expression, softness of voice and gentle touch of the animal.
- Explain what you are finding in a way that is intelligible for that particular client.
- Avoid using emotive words like 'cancer'. It is kinder to say 'lump' or 'growth'. The client's pre-knowledge may depend on traumatic personal family experience, especially with cancer.
- Provide time. Except in absolute crisis, owners should not be asked to make decisions about euthanasia when they are still stunned by hearing of the possible severity of the situation. The vet's judgement also should not be made hurriedly without taking measures to confirm a tentative diagnosis. Owners must be clear headed, well informed and left knowing that they have not been rushed into decisions which may later be regretted.

Options for providing time

There are two options depending on the situation.

(a) You may say that you would like to keep the animal in for a few hours in order to make a more detailed examination. If the animal is critical, at least this gives a short time for adjustment to bad news, and for informing the family.

(b) Admit the animal for further examination and possible tests (advise about costs). Delay admission for some minutes, telling the owner that you need to prepare a bed for (Tibby). This gives owners valuable time with an animal that may be nearing the end of its life.

This is especially important when owners do not realise just how ill the animal is.

- However, if you think the animal may die overnight, take option (a). It is very distressing for owners to think the animal died alone in a kennel.
- Take samples for tests and let owners take the animal home with some palliative or interim treatment (painkillers if necessary).

Next meeting
- **Review** what you found at the first examination and give any new information from test results.
- **Check** for understanding, using diagrams and analogies (see Section 1.2).
- People forget a lot of what they hear, especially when it is unexpected and unwelcome.
- **Show consideration,** especially when you are intimating that the outlook is poor. Show the owner that you care, by your tone of voice and the way you look at them. Always refer to the animal by its name, not 'the dog' or 'the cat'.
- Explain the situation by speaking slowly, allowing pauses for questions and assimilation of information. Consider if you can offer any realistic hope and whether there are options other than euthanasia. Always inform clients, making sure that they have heard you, about what the costs of 'options' might be in terms of the well-being of the animal, the strain on the family, and the financial costs. Often a client will say 'I do not care what it costs' without having a notion of what is involved.
- **Be prepared** for owners' reaction to bad news. It may be stark disbelief and denial, stunned shock, anger, tears, embarrassment, occasionally even hysteria. Some clients are likely to become defensive, even hostile.

Remember that when people are in shock and denial it is likely that they will not hear things or will misunderstand what has been said. Be as clear and supportive as possible, maybe putting things in writing for them to show their families.

Never make exact predictions about life expectancy
However, clients do press for more information. It often helps a client whose animal has a terminal problem, e.g. heart failure, to give a broad prediction (e.g. weeks against months). If you keep it vague and open, at least you give people a small handle to hold onto. If the animal lives longer, the owner often quotes this to you.

If you remain 'broad shouldered' about such comments the owner may feel they have 'beaten' the disease, even when the animal subsequently dies. Even if the death comes sooner than expected, it is still better to have given them some idea, as long as the communication was good and they realised the impossibility of accuracy.

Encourage questions. Listen to their ideas, fears and doubts. Acknowledge by your body language and words, that you are aware of their distress. Enquire about the rest of the family, especially any children. What are their views?

Comment

Do not blame an anxious owner: caring owners usually carry a lot of guilt concerning their animals' illnesses and death. Even when you feel that they have been negligent in some way do not compound their distress by making them feel even more guilty.

For vets who are so tuned in to animals' health and well-being, it is upsetting to have an animal presented (which obviously should have been brought in earlier) in the mid or later stages of terminal illness.

If an owner is obviously surprised and upset when advised of the severity of the condition, do not berate them or say 'if only you'd brought him in sooner'. It may be that:

- An underlying condition had suddenly worsened.
- There had been serious distraction, such as family illness, death, separation.
- The family were fearful that the vet would advise euthanasia at an earlier stage.

Shock

The shock of bad news makes logical thinking difficult. If irrevocable decisions are made at that time, there is almost bound to be devastating doubt and self-recrimination afterwards. If possible, give owners a chance to assimilate the information, and to contact family members. Other people who care about the animal may be devastated if they have not been consulted, and had no opportunity to say 'goodbye'. This leads to anger and blaming rather than mutual support.

A vet says:

I write to the children explaining why I helped their animal companion to die peacefully. This has been found to be very helpful and much appreciated by parents who report that they believe this has prevented the children from blaming them – a very common reaction. Letters have also been sent to spouses who did not attend the surgery.

Anaesthetic death of apparently healthy animals

Always inform owners about possible risks before giving deep sedation or anaesthetics

- The death of healthy animals undergoing operational procedures is devastating for all concerned.
- The vet should contact owners immediately. They will probably sense something is wrong by your tone of voice. Tell them what happened. Try to give some explanation (there may have been some pathology that did not show up clinically) or be frank that these sad unexplained deaths do happen, even to people with all the best equipment available.
- Be prepared for long silences while they adjust to the news.
- Give them time to decide about the body.
- Convey how sad you are, without apologising.
- The staff are quickly drawn in. They feel awful, but will have to be prepared to answer phone calls from the owners who will probably have questions about why it happened.
- The staff have a loyalty to the practice and at the same time need to be sensitive and caring to the owners. Coach them in what they are to say and recognize the difficulty everyone is experiencing.
- Have a staff meeting so that everyone can discuss the situation and share feelings.
- Do not send a bill.
- Do send a personal letter, expressing the sadness of all the staff.

WHEN OWNERS MAY HAVE HAD SOME PREPARATION

When there is a serious deterioration of an in-patient

Have the necessary telephone numbers where the owner can be contacted (and other family numbers).

Find out
Which staff member has been dealing most closely with the case or who has best rapport with the client.

Action
It is essential to **contact the owner immediately.**

Who phones?
- The most appropriate person should phone and suggest the owner should come in, saying that the animal's condition is worrying or things have taken a change for the worse.
- If possible avoid **talking about euthanasia over the phone.** Suggest other family members may want to come in as well.
- If you contact an answer phone, just leave a message, asking them to get in touch with the surgery immediately.

Comment
If the animal does die, or is euthanased, the family have a right, if not a need, to be there.

- Phone the owner immediately if an animal's condition deteriorates, or it dies.
- If it dies overnight, phone first thing in the morning. Some vets will actually visit the owners to break the bad news, especially when the death has been unexpected. Owners really appreciate that.
- The cause of death should be explained; people need to know 'why'.
- Owners often ask for details. What time did it die? Was the death peaceful? It certainly helps if you can say that someone was with the animal, or someone had been comforting it before it 'slipped away'.
- The owner may want to see the body. Empty the bladder to avoid mess.
- Always make the body look peaceful; some vets use cardboard ready-made coffins.
- Do not place the body in the freezer until you are certain the owner does not want to view it.
- If you do put it in a freezer, still make the animal look comfortable and position the legs to facilitate burial or placement in body bag (the owner may decide to take the body after all).

When incurable problems are found during laparotomy

Always have emergency contact numbers before doing laparotomies, especially exploratory.

Provide for an action plan in case of euthanasia decisions. This should be discussed beforehand. Some owners would want to be with their animal before and during euthanasia; others prefer to come in after the death.

Make immediate contact
On finding a severe problem situation, contact the owner immediately so that they can have the choice to be there during euthanasia (which in anaesthetised animals cannot be deferred for long).

Reducing client stress
• The operating room may be intimidating to owners.
• Move the animal and anaesthetic trolley to a consulting room.
• Cover the wound and clean up any blood.
• Make the animal look natural and peaceful.

3

Helping clients through decision making

GENERAL INFORMATION FOR HELPING WITH DECISIONS INVOLVING POSSIBLE EUTHANASIA FOR REASONS OF ILL HEALTH OR INJURY:

- Because euthanasia exists as an alternative to natural death, owners are frequently faced with decisions they are totally unprepared to make.
- Over half the deaths of animals under veterinary care are as a result of euthanasia, and the implications for each imposed death must be carefully considered.
- Be familiar with the average life spans of all pets and be conservative in quoting upper limits.
- Never be hasty with euthanasia decisions. Unless an animal is so severely injured or in such agony that there is no choice, always give an animal a chance to recover.
- A common source of anxiety following animal death is the uncertainty or regret about choices which were made. People may feel that they have been pressurised, or rushed, or that they had been too confused or upset to question the vet's recommendations.
- Although the decision is ultimately the owner's, obviously the vet's opinion has great influence.
- The vet's responsibility is to balance the welfare of the animal and the needs of the owner.

Find out
Find out the following details about the owner's situation:
- What is their relationship with the animal? Is it 'my baby', 'one of the family', 'best friend'? (Occasionally owners are ambivalent and there are some who do not care strongly at all.)
- Do they assume responsibility, and guilt, for anything that 'goes wrong' with their animal?

- Do they need to feel that they have done everything possible to help their animal?
- Would they feel more reassured to have a second opinion (sometimes if only to confirm poor prognosis)? Most owners are happy to have a second opinion arranged within the practice. You can also offer to review the animal's case with the other practice vets, i.e. arrange a case discussion. (Note: It is distressing for a client if the second opinion conflicts with what they have been told already, so care should be taken by both parties to co-operate in reaching a consensus.)
- Are they reluctant to choose euthanasia even when they feel they just cannot cope with the nursing, or watching their sick animal? This is especially difficult in central nervous system cases where the animal's actions can be very distressing. Most owners are grateful for the offer of hospitalisation.
- Do they require 'permission' to consider their own needs?

Action
- **Be supportive** of owners, acknowledging how difficult all this must be for them.
- **Educate** owners; in order to prepare themselves for the possibility of death, the owners need to understand the condition and options for therapy.
- Explain, using familiar terms, maybe drawing diagrams to illustrate.
- Avoid ambiguity, like 'put down' or 'put to sleep'. This is especially important with children who may be afraid to go to sleep. Do not use the words 'destroy' or 'bump'.
- **Check for understanding.** Encourage questions and discussion of anxieties.
- **Prepare** owners. During supportive care in severe illness, stress quality of life and introduce the possibility of 'helping to die' as an option in a therapeutic plan. Do not be reluctant to talk about death while there is the option of living. When describing what is available, compare short-term discomfort with long-term outlook.
- **Warning!** Never make predictions one way or another.

In making decisions about prolonging or ending life, the following need to be considered:

The animal's character; does it have a lot of courage and a will to live?

The animal's physical and mental well-being. Has it:

- Lost the ability to get up and move around without assistance?
- Lost interest in going outside for walks, or being sociable?
- Become distressed, and anxious, especially if left alone? Is it whining for attention?

The owner's ability to cope with a seriously ill animal
- Physically, with demands of nursing care and attention.
- Financially, if there is no insurance cover, to make sure they know the probable cost.
- Emotionally with the ups and downs of therapy, and possible deterioration.

Indicators from the animal
- Pain: is the animal obviously feeling pain which cannot be alleviated?
- Suffering: is the animal suffering, physically or mentally? You may have to explain that suffering does not have to involve pain.
- Are there some good days and some bad? Are the bad days increasing?

Quality of life
Has the animal:

- Lost control of defecation and urination?
- Difficulty in breathing?
- Lost interest in eating and drinking?

Does the owner have support from other family members?
Sometimes people are under a lot of pressure from others, family, friends or neighbours, who pass negative comments. Sometimes vets are asked to provide letters explaining the condition, for owners to show to those who pass comments.

Will the owner have continuing support from the practice?
This question is up to you and the owner needs to be reassured about this. If owners choose to embark on a long-term therapy program, the vet must be prepared to support them emotionally through the illness, as well as caring for the animal medically.

Guide, do not pressurize, owners into decisions. If they ask 'What would you do?', be gently honest, while emphasizing that it has to be their decision. Try and find out what they really want, and support them in that (as long as the welfare of the animal is not jeopardized).

Encourage clients to involve the family in decisions, writing down points they could discuss.

Warn clients that even though euthanasia can be the kindest action, feeling guilty about considering euthanasia is natural and almost inevitable.

Check points
- Were the client's feelings acknowledged?
- Was the welfare of the animal always considered?
- Was it given 'a chance' to recover?
- Did the client understand the medical condition?
- Were the therapeutic options explained and understood?
- Was the client encouraged to ask questions and to express concerns?
- Did the client feel supported in the final decision and reassured that it was the right one for them?

If the decision is for euthanasia, some vets schedule a time for pre-euthanasia discussion without the animal being present.

This gives owners time to think about things and to make plans with a clearer mind.

Clients' complaints about decision making
- They did not understand what was the matter with their animal or why it died.
- They were unsure about the choice of treatment.
- They felt stupid and were not given the opportunity to ask questions.
- They thought the treatment would keep their dog alive for another year, but it died in a few weeks.
- They felt pressurized into a decision they regretted later.
- Seeing different vets added to the confusion over diagnosis, prognosis and treatment.

Fear is diminished when we give something a name. By simply naming it we take possession of it.

(from *An Evil Cradling* by Brian Keenan)

4

Pre-euthanasia discussion

Many vets encourage clients to come to the surgery at a quiet time, without the animal, for an informal talk about an impending euthanasia.

Think
- This discussion gives the client a chance to make plans and prepare for dealing with the euthanasia in a way they will not regret later.
- This important interview should be conducted with sensitivity to the client's perceptions.
- This is usually considered as being part of the service, not an extra expense for the client.

Find out
Establish the details of the case and the basis for the decision to euthanase.

Action
- Sit down with the client, giving good attention.
- Acknowledge how difficult this must be, and be caring and supportive in your approach.
- Review the recent course of events, leading up to the decision for euthanasia.
- Take time for last-minute uncertainties and anxieties.
- Ensure that this is what the client still wants and be reassuring that this is the kindest thing they can do for (name the animal).

Options
Clarify options to consider

- **Where?** Home based which is easier on the client and the animal, or at surgery, which has advantages for the vet.
- **By whom?** Obviously it is best done by someone with whom both animal and owner are comfortable.

- **When?** ASAP once the decision is made and at a time when the preferred vet is available.
- **Who should be present?** Do the owner and other family members want to be there? As long as things go smoothly, owners feel good about having stayed. If things go wrong, they are left with painful memories. If children are to be present, they should know what to expect.
- **What will happen?** This is an opportunity to explain the procedure. That an anaesthetic solution will be injected into a vein, that the animal will become unconscious and die very quickly. If owners are not prepared, the suddenness may be shocking. Prepare them about the options for sedation or the possible use of other injection sites. You might inform them that the eyes will remain open, there may be a sudden gasp or sigh, and the muscles may twitch. There may be also a relaxing of body sphincters. Some vets prefer to give these final details at the time of euthanasia or just at the end.
- **How might they themselves react?** It is helpful for owners to be prepared about the sort of reaction they might have. Many are unprepared for the intensity of their feelings.

Aftercare of the body
It is easier to discuss this without the animal present, and while owners are relatively calm. Along with making plans for the body, some owners will want to know about the activities or rituals that other people have found helpful, especially where children are involved.

Demonstrate an appropriate attitude
Clients have commented on the importance of their vet's openness and kindness while discussing these potentially upsetting things. Qualities in a vet that give clients a feeling of being held, understood and looked after are: being honest, open, and at ease with personal and other people's emotions. Being trusting of their vets will help clients have confidence to face the procedures that will follow. Avoid being difficult or hesitant, acting cold, or embarrassed, or withdrawing at signs of emotions. Also avoid being over emotional; clients should not have to worry about the vet's ability to cope. This does not mean you should not get sad or even watery eyed. Just be controlled in it.

5

The process of euthanasia

Euthanasia decisions have been agreed upon. In some cases, a pre-euthanasia discussion has taken place. All concerned, vets, nurses and staff should be prepared for coping with anxious and distressed clients (alerted by messages about scheduled euthanasias on staff notice board).

Never become casual about euthanasia.

- For the vet, though it is part of the job, it can be either one of the most rewarding or the most stressful aspects of the practice.
- For the animal, it is the end of its life and it should be a peaceful passing.
- For the owner, it may be a significant life event, maybe the most difficult experience they have ever had to face. (A dentist said to a friend, 'It was the worst day of my life. I sat looking at Bonnie and thinking, today I am going to take my best pal to be killed!')

The way a practice deals with euthanasia will probably determine the client's enduring attitude to the vet, the practice, and to the death itself.

CLINIC-BASED EUTHANASIA

Find out
- If the owner has been to a pre-euthanasia discussion.
- If arrangements have been made so that the owner does not have long to wait and preferably not in the area with other clients. Sometimes consultations run late, so it is best if appointments can be made before the others or out of usual hours.
- If all staff are aware of the impending euthanasia.

Action
- Ensure that everyone acts sensitively and speaks kindly to the animal, using its name.

- There should be no laughter or joking in the background.
- Avoid anything which may increase anxiety about the decision e.g. making cheery comments like, 'Smokey is looking a bit brighter today!'. (It sometimes happens that an animal momentarily perks up just at the time when all the final plans have been made, undermining the owner's resolve).
- If it is considered necessary to have a signed consent from that particular client, present the consent form in a sensitive manner, checking for understanding and then acknowledging the difficulty of having to sign that form.

Confirm the client's decision whether or not to stay during euthanasia. Explain that while you are attending to the animal all your concentration will have to be focused on what you are doing and that no one will be free to attend to their needs. If they think they cannot be supportive to the animal, or cannot cope, give them a chance to change their mind.

One vet says:

I have never experienced an owner causing worry to an animal during euthanasia. If they are unsure about staying, they can always start by staying, then leave if they cannot cope.

What about children?
If a child really wishes to be there when their pet dies, the final decision rests with the parents and the vet, depending on both age and emotional maturity of the child, and the possibility of difficulties with the procedure.

Speak to the child alone and check that they really do want to attend and are not just trying to please. Explain the procedure, check for understanding. Make sure they know about the agonal gasp.

If children are present, it is vitally important that everything goes smoothly, so that the child is not left with a difficult memory. Someone should be able to be there to comfort the child. A potentially less stressful option is for the child to come in with the animal, give it a cuddle, go out and wait while the injection is being given, and then come in again to say goodbye.

Client-present euthanasia

Think
While witnessing a euthanasia an owner will have a heightened sensitivity to everything that happens. Everything that is said or done becomes MAGNIFIED and highly significant. Years of good practice

and good client relationships will be discounted if the death has been unsatisfactory.

Familiar vet
Ideally euthanasia should be performed by a vet who has treated the animal and has a good relationship with both it and the client. If this is impossible, the client should be informed. Every effort should be made to have an attending nurse with whom the client has built up a rapport.

Find out
Is the room supplied with two chairs (or more if several people attending), a box of tissues, a fleece or mat for sliding under the animal and some absorbent wipes, a blanket or cover of some sort if the owner has not brought one?

Some vets have a large mat or a coloured fleece (fleece comes in various sizes and colours; the blue is a favourite) for performing euthanasia on the floor, if clients wish to sit with their larger dogs. (Some older clients cannot manage that, of course.)

A vet unfamiliar with the animal should review any case records, and know about the circumstances and details, especially the name of the owner and name and sex of the animal. Check the age of the animal again. Owners will often ask 'Was Pepe's lifespan normal for his breed?'.

Action
- Arrange that there should be no interruptions during euthanasia. Turn off any pagers.
- Reassure the owner that you know this has been a tough decision, but they are doing the kindest thing they can.
- Explain the procedure: 'We'll just clip a little hair so we can see the vein better.' 'He'll just feel a little pinprick when he gets the injection of concentrated anaesthetic. Then he'll start to take a few deep breaths as he becomes unconscious.' Prepare them for the rapid change from life to death; warn them that there may be a few reflex gasps and that the eyes will remain open.
- Show the owner where to stand (or sit if on the floor). Advise them about supporting the animal's head (they are often taken unaware by the speed of the drugs' action). Say that it would be helpful if they could stroke and talk to the animal while you induce anaesthesia.
- Tell them that their voice and touch will comfort the animal as it dies (see Comment).

- Giving this support to their animal instead of just being a witness to the death helps owners to cope and lessens their guilt.
- Discourage owners who want to hold the animal themselves, instead of letting the nurse restrain it. Explain tactfully that the animal would prefer the owner to be in front where it can see them.

The death
- Calm the animal, treating it gently and stroking it. After making the injection, speak to the animal softly by name as it dies and carefully slip it down into a comfortable looking position.
- Use the short time before the heart and respirations stop to tidy the animal, remove syringes, needles, scissors, wipe away any hair clippings and blood, and put absorbent material in place in case of sphincter relaxation.
- Warn again about that possibility and of agonal gasp and muscle twitching after death. This might have been explained in a pre-euthanasia discussion, but owners may need reminding. Some vets feel that it is better not to give such details in the pre-dis-cussion, but to wait until the actual time of euthanasia (too much information at a time will not be heard).
- If the owner is holding the animal on their lap, provide them with a thick towel and wipes, warning them that they may get wet, or worse.
- Confirm with a stethoscope that the heart has stopped beating (explaining that this is routine). Then say whatever seems appro-priate for the owner, something like, *'That's it, she's peaceful now'*. It is a gentle way of saying the animal is dead and also reinforces the fact that the death has come as a relief for the pet.
- Make sure the animal looks peaceful, maybe covering the body with a small blanket, leaving the head out.

Then give full attention to the owner.

Comment
How one vet explains the different stages to the owner:

> *She is feeling very sleepy now but is still aware of you. If you want, stroke her and talk to her.*
> *She has lost consciousness now and is not aware of anything. Her heart is very weak now.*

This vet prefers to say 'She's passed over' as this seems softer and gentler.

Advantages of owner being present
For the client:

- Not having to imagine what may have happened.
- Reassurance that the animal had a good death.
- Knowing that they had held and comforted their animal as it was dying. That although it was difficult for them, it was their last gift to the animal. 'She was always there for me and I promised her that I would always be there for her.' 'She died in my arms, I could not have let her die alone.' 'It was so peaceful and everyone was so kind to both of us.'
- In general, people who stay seem to have fewer problems afterwards, both in accepting the death and coping with their loss.

For the vet:

- If everything goes well, close bonds are made with the client.
- There may be a sense of deep satisfaction, of having helped and made a difference

Disadvantages of owner being present
It is potentially more stressful for the vet and staff, requiring more time and attention to detail. If things go wrong, it can be devastating for owners and very difficult for the vet.

Some complaints from clients
- The staff were joking about something and I felt like shouting at them.
- I was left in a waiting room full of other people and someone asked me why we were in.
- The 'wrong' vet, who did not even know us, was on duty, instead of the one we had made arrangements with.
- My old dog was walking slowly and the vet seemed impatient and dragged him roughly.
- The vet never spoke a word to the dog the whole time.
- My dog was frightened and started to struggle, then as the vet tried to give him the injection, he started screaming. The vet seemed angry.
- I'll never forget the fear in his eyes. That look was still there after he was dead. His eyes were wide open in fright (owner had not been warned about the eyes staying open).
- I thought he was dead, then he was breathing again. I did not know what was happening.
- The vet was good enough I guess, but cold. She did not seem to care about me or my Tibbie.

The mechanics of the procedure

Most vets have their own ways of managing euthanasias, and have developed their own personal strategies for dealing with difficult ones. The condition of the animal, the composure and preference of the owner and the confidence and competence of the vet are deciding factors.

It is important that the strategy used should be explained to the owner in a confident and composed manner, acknowledging difficulty in a way that implies control and compassion.

People accept things more readily if they understand what is happening and why.

Procedures for dealing with potentially difficult situations

Animals with poor blood pressure/fragile veins

- Shave both forelimbs, explaining to the owner: 'Topsy's old, her blood pressure is poor and her veins are fragile. So we're preparing both veins and we'll use the one that looks best. If we have any problems with one, the other leg is ready.' This lets them know what you are doing and alerts them to the fact that there may be problems.
- If there is difficulty getting into a vein, take the animal into a prep room and insert an intravenous line, instead of having to make several attempts in front of the owner. When the animal is returned, the owner may be able to hold it while the injection is being made. If the femoral vein is used, the owner may cradle the animal's body.

Animals that are nervous, frightened and jumpy

A final struggle is very upsetting for the owners, and animals should not have to die in fear.

- Speak to the animal in a calm, gentle manner.
- Rubbing a local anaesthetic cream into the injection site (as used to facilitate intravenous injection in children) can be useful with sensitive animals but needs time to take effect.
- Giving a tranquilliser like acepromazine maleate (ACP) will help the animal relax. After sedating the animal, let the owner stay until the animal loses awareness. Explain that sedation means that there is no discomfort, but that a drop in blood pressure makes getting into the veins even more difficult. An alternative parenteral site may need to be used, and the owner may prefer to go out for a few minutes and then return to be with the animal

while it is dying. Explain that the procedure takes a few minutes longer than the intravenous injection.

Aggressive or dangerous animals
- Human safety is paramount. If anyone gets hurt in your surgery, you are responsible (even if the owner is bitten by his own dog!). The comfort and well-being of the animal must also be considered. However frustrating, never show anger or frustration towards an animal that is being euthanased.
- ACP may not be an adequate tranquilliser; consider Medetomidine or Xylazine. Very difficult animals may require large doses, adding considerable cost to the procedure.
- Keep a full set of muzzles. Explain to the owner 'Tyson has a record of trying to bite his vet, so he needs to wear a muzzle just until the solution takes effect. It is a very comfortable muzzle'. A big dog wearing a basket muzzle can give a painful head butt so he needs good restraint of the head. (Some vets will not use muzzles and find sedation preferable).
- Always remove the muzzle as soon as possible and say to the owner you regret that 'Tyson' had to wear it.
- In some cases a tape muzzle may be sufficient; but do not take chances. Before applying it, explain to the owner that it will not restrict the breathing.

Animals which are fitting
This can be very difficult and owners may be very distressed:

- Fitting cats can be given intrahepatic pentabarbitone sodium, which acts quickly.
- Dogs can be given medetomidine, though some minutes will be required to take effect. Once the animal is relaxed the intravenous injection should be possible.
- It helps owners to see their animals resting and looking peaceful again.
- They may need explanations about fitting, and assurances that their animal was not aware of anything.

Alternative parenteral routes
Clients sometimes have difficulty with the idea of injections where the needle goes into the body (not 'on the surface'). Some of these routes are more acceptable than others.

- Intracardiac injections are distressing for owners to witness but can result in immediate death. If there is difficulty with the injection and intrathoracic leakage, there can be great pain.
- Intraperitoneal injections are painless, but take time. Animals, especially cats, may become distressed, and even frantic, as their control starts to go. When they are held and comforted as they lose consciousness, then the death is peaceful.
- Intrahepatic route for cats is quick and seems to be painless. Cats rarely notice the injection and lose consciousness in about 2 minutes. A cat can sit on an owner's lap while being injected. Many clients prefer this route, as do nurses, for no shaving of legs or restraint is necessary. It is important to use more of the solution (about 10 ml) than for intravenous injection.
- Intrarenal injections may cause more discomfort than hepatic, but can be very quick and successful in thin cats.

Clients not wishing to witness euthanasia

- They may ask a friend or relative to be present instead. This is a stressful task for them, and they need to be prepared and supported in the same way as the owner. It is important that they tell the owner that the death was peaceful.
- When owners do not want to stay during euthanasia, be supportive of their decision.
- Explain the procedure and reassure them it will be painless and peaceful.
- Name the attending nurse and say that she will be stroking, caressing and talking to the animal.
- Say that it will be performed immediately, unless a sedative is required, and if so, explain.
- Reassure them about euthanasia being the right course of action.
- Give them the option of coming in afterwards for a last goodbye. This helps them to accept that the animal has really died.
- It comforts them to see their pet is looking peaceful, especially if it had been distressed in life.

If the owners want to leave, and do not want to come back in to see their animal, reassure them (as above) and make sure they have chosen their option for disposing of the body.

You can give them sheets with information on pet loss and support. Ring them shortly after they have reached home to reassure them that the euthanasia has been done and that the animal is at rest, or you might want to write a note to tell them that the death was peaceful.

FOLLOWING DEATH

Immediately after euthanasia or death

Attend to the owner, after arranging the dead animal in a comfortable looking position, with an absorbent pad beneath and a drape or blanket over the back, possibly with a folded pillow under the head.

This is a valuable time for establishing a continuing relationship with your client.

Make your attention appropriate to the owner's needs.

Some people are surprized by the power of their own emotions. Be prepared for a range of emotional reactions: sobbing, stunned disbelief, denial, hysteria, anger, quiet floods of tears, guilt and even embarrassment at 'making a spectacle', especially for men when they 'break down' in front of women.

Be prepared, if it seems appropriate, to give clients information about grief reactions and available support.

Find out

- If they want a few minutes alone to say their last goodbye or to have a cry in private.
- If they want you to be there with them for a few minutes.
- If they just want to leave (preferably by an exit other than the waiting room).

Action

- If the owner wants privacy, go out of the room, telling them when you will be back. (Remove any bottles and syringes.)
- When owners are crying, distressed or seem very upset, pass them a tissue (letting them know it is OK to cry). Offer them a seat. You may even sit with them for a few minutes.
- If clients are embarrassed about being upset, reassure them it is normal and you would be more worried about them if they were not.
- Offer whatever support seems appropriate, maybe a comforting touch, an arm around the shoulder or even a hug. Use your judgement; this can be tricky with opposite sexes!
- Be receptive if they want to talk about their animal or even about previous losses. (Very often other losses will surface at this time, and it is important to listen and acknowledge what they are telling you). This is time very well spent. Clients remember such support with gratitude.

- Acknowledging their sadness, reassure them that it is appropriate to feel like that when they have lost something so precious, that they do not need to be afraid or embarrassed about feeling bad. Let them know that they are not alone and that most people who lose a loved animal feel much the same.
- Warn them that as well as feeling sad, many people tend to feel some degree of guilt, and that is also normal, in fact almost inevitable.
- Owners may wish to reminisce about happy times and tell funny stories about their pets. It helps them to be listened to and it is sometimes a relief for them to know it is OK to be smiling as well as crying.
- If a client does not seem too upset, do not assume that they do not care. Many people are not comfortable showing their feelings. They need and appreciate privacy. Avoid interventions that break their composure. This must be respected. However, even though you are restrained with your words, you can still show that you are caring by the way you handle the animal's body, and by subtle signs, by your gentleness and tone of voice.
- It might be that the death comes as a relief to an owner who has suffered along with an animal during all of the nursing and care. So along with sadness, there may be gratitude that it is all over. (There may even be guilt caused by the recognition of feelings of relief.)
- Arrangements for the body will need to be discussed. Hopefully, this will have been arranged beforehand. If not, it needs to be broached sensitively. Avoid words like 'dispose', 'incinerate', etc. If the client leaves the body, the last impression should be peaceful.
- If the owner is very distressed, settle them in a quiet spot, maybe with a cup of tea, before they leave the surgery. This is especially important if they are driving.
- Offer to call a friend or a taxi. In some cases it is even appropriate for a staff member to take them home (and make them a cup of tea!).

As the clients leave
- You may want to reassure them that they did the 'right thing', e.g. something like 'You gave him a wonderful life, and then helped him through right to the end. It was the best gift you could give him.'
- If you say, 'I know **we made the right decision**', you are sharing the responsibility and it helps absolve their guilt.

- If they leave by a different exit, accompany them so that they do not get lost and need to ask someone the way out.

Comment
One vet describes his procedure following euthanasia:

> *I explain to the owner that when the animal dies, first the breathing stops and then the heart. After giving the injection, I absent myself by going to get a stethoscope, allowing the owners some private space. Then I come back, check there is no heartbeat and say 'he's gone' or 'it is all over now'. I do not actually leave the room then because it might appear as if I'm no longer interested. They may want to ask a question or be reassured. I do try and merge with the background, so the owners feel less inhibited and can say goodbye however they want to.*

Some owners want minimal involvement with anything after the death; others want to plan every detail.

Collars
Small things can have considerable significance.

- If the body is being left at the surgery, ask 'Would you like him just to keep his collar on, or would you like to take it home?'.
- Sometimes people like to leave the collar on but keep the name tag. Children may like to put the tag somewhere special, with their small treasures.
- Do not just say, 'Do you want the collar?'. To some, this is disrespectful to the animal.
- It is important to clarify just what their wishes are. Some clients phone up days after expecting to still be able to change their mind and have the collar back.

The body
Always handle the body gently and with respect, whether the client is taking or leaving it.
Things which have given comfort to clients who are leaving the body:

- Seeing the animal looking so tranquil.
- Taking a Polaroid photograph. Dead animals look so peaceful, it is good to save that last impression.
- Asking the client if they would like to save a tuft of hair.
- Asking the client if they would like to have a paw print made. These can be made with ordinary ink on A4 paper. If the spot is

hairy, clip out a little hair for a clearer print. Some practices make plaster paw prints as well.

If the client is taking the animal home
- Express the bladder before wrapping the body in a blanket or something the client has supplied. Leave the head out.
- Never put in a plastic bag. Slip a plastic sheet or folded bag under the body in case of sphincter relaxation, explaining your reasons.
- Warn the owner that there may be a little muscle twitching and ask them to arrange the body in the desired position for burial before rigor mortis sets in.

Uncaring owners
- These are very different from, and not to be confused with, owners who just do not want to show emotions.
- Some people who are not greatly attached to an animal may have no feelings of regret or sadness.
- There are a few people who actively dislike an animal which they have been looking after.
- You should be able to tell by their manner with the animal and your own sensitivity.
- In these cases, expectations of an emotional response are not appreciated by the owners. (It is usually the vet staff who are sad, upset and angry at their uncaring attitude.)

The bill
- If the client is unknown to the practice, it is important to collect the fee before the euthanasia, saying something like, 'It is easier for you if we square up the bill now'.
- Otherwise, ask what the client wants. Some prefer to pay in advance, others later. It is best not done at the time of the euthanasia unless they want to 'get it over with'. If so, allow them to pay in the consulting room, not at the main desk.
- When making out a hand-written bill, write 'veterinary services provided'. Avoid using the terms 'euthanasia' or 'disposal'. Computer invoices will be programmed to include the word euthanasia, so it cannot be avoided.
- If the bill is sent out later, add a wee note as well so it does not seem so harsh.
- Never send the bill at the same time as a condolence card!

Things that are helpful
- Showing respect for the body.

- Respecting the clients' need for company or for privacy.
- Treating clients with kindness. Giving them the support they need.
- Being there for clients who want to talk, even though it is for a short time.
- Being familiar with signs of grief and at ease with other people's emotions.
- Being comfortable with your own emotions, so that you can react appropriately.
- Acknowledging their loss, 'normalising' their grief.
- Being empathic and honest.
- Reassuring that 'if it had been me, I'd have done the same'.

Things to avoid
- Being patronizing and over-protective when it is not appropriate.
- Appearing to be cold and clinical.
- Being detached to the point of appearing not to care.
- Being so diffident, or hesitant, that the client does not have confidence in your judgement.
- Being so emotional that the client has to be the strong one.
- Saying things like 'Time is a great healer'; 'You'll soon feel better'; 'I feel just as badly as you do'; 'I know just how you feel'; 'We just have to accept that animals have a shorter life than us'; 'I know a lovely (puppy, cat) that is looking for a home'.

Continuing client support

Almost all clients appreciate receiving some sort of personal letter or card after a loved animal's death.

In a private communication, Sir Chris Bonnington writes:

Our Lab, Bella, became ill and we took her to the vet hospital and had to leave her there for tests. She was diagnosed as having cancer and the vet phoned to say it had gone too far and it would be kinder to put her down. Since she was already in the hospital, we asked her to give the injection.

A few days later we had a lovely letter from the vet who had looked after her, telling us how fond she had been of Bella, how she had given her a cuddle before injecting her, and that she had died peacefully. They also sent Bella's ashes back in a little wooden casket. The sensitivity and kindness of that vet and the staff of the hospital was a great consolation to us.

Condolence cards
A condolence card or letter should be sent a day or two after the death. This should commemorate the animal in some way, possibly with a personal reminiscence. It should contain reassurances that the death was peaceful if the owners were not present, and acknowledge that this must be a sad time for them, or whatever is appropriate.

For clients known to be grieving
Vets and clinic staff may be the only people who appreciate the impact of animal death on their clients' lives. Any follow up support is usually greatly appreciated.

Find out
Find out if staff are aware of the client's home circumstances and involve them in a follow up policy.

Action
- Send a condolence card.
- Offer helpful leaflets or information sheets. Some practices give all their clients their own 'pet loss support leaflets' (also sending them to clients who notify the practice that their animals have died).
- Have available BSAVA leaflets and SCAS/Blue Cross information about Befrienders.
- Make phone calls. When clients who are known to be living alone have appeared to be devastated by a death, it is good practice to give them a ring in the next few days. This lets them know someone is thinking about them, and usually brings them comfort. Vets sometimes forget what an important role they have had in some people's lives.
- Suggest reading material; this is useful for emphasising the shared aspects of grieving for pets. The surgery should make a reading list available, and may even have books for lending to adults and children.
- Answer questions. Vets can offer clients assistance with questions that might be troubling them. Closure is important and sometimes little uncertainties can get in the way of resolving grief.
- Provide details of groups or individuals who might give further help with emotional support or counselling. Some social workers or ministers who have experienced pet loss may be known to the practice.
- Some practices may get involved in local pet loss support groups.

- There are training courses for nurses who are interested in learning more about supporting clients through animal death.
- When offering support it is important not to encourage the client to become dependent upon you. This does a dis-service to the client as well as creating a problem with the invasion of your personal life.
- Unless unusual circumstances prevail, vets should limit their support and help to issues about animal loss. Boundaries need to be established and respected.

Euthanasia checklist

Some euthanasias seem to go more smoothly than others and many owners, in spite of their sadness, express deep gratitude to the vet staff for 'being so kind'. This is a very rewarding aspect of the practice, and it is useful to reflect on the factors which may influence your clients' perceptions.

Before
- Where possible, was the owner given an opportunity to adjust to receiving 'bad news'?
- Was the owner fully taking in what was being said?
- Did the owner understand the diagnoses, the treatment of the animal?
- Where appropriate, had consideration been given to other alternatives?
- Was the animal given a reasonable chance?
- Was the owner encouraged to ask questions?
- Was the owner left feeling reassured that everything possible was being done (in the interest of both themselves and their animal)?
- Was consideration given to the feelings and opinions of other family members, especially children?
- Was there an opportunity for a pre-euthanasia discussion?

Euthanasia
- Did everyone in the family have a chance to say goodbye?
- Was the owner given the choice to have the animal euthanised at home?
- If performed at the surgery, were staff alerted and prepared for the owner's situation?
- Was the owner given the opportunity to stay with the animal?
- If they did stay, were they told what to expect (last gasp, etc.)?

- Were arrangements made so that the owner had some privacy before and after the euthanasia?
- Was the procedure successful? Was the death painless and peaceful?
- Was there any attempt to make the dead animal look comfortable and at peace?
- If the owner did not stay were they offered the chance to come in afterwards?
- In either case were they allowed to have a moment's privacy to say goodbye?
- Were both the animal and owner treated with sensitivity and kindness by all the staff involved?

After euthanasia
- Was the body treated with respect?
- Was the body disposed of in a way that the owner wished? Had options been discussed?
- Was the owner given consideration and support?
- Was there anything that seemed to cause extra concern or distress?
- Were all the staff supportive? Was any follow up considered to be appropriate?

What about feelings
- What did the owner seem to be experiencing?
- How were you left feeling about your part in the procedure?
- How were the rest of the staff reacting?

Was there any feedback from the clients?

OPTIONS FOR THE BODY

Ideally this will have been discussed and arranged at a time when the owner is not so confused that they cannot make a clear and balanced decision.

As with human death, there are some people who get comfort by providing an elaborate burial, whereas others want to keep it as simple possible.

The practice should have details of:

- The options for dealing with animals' bodies.
- Detailed information about local services and the approximate costs involved.

Leave body for the practice to make arrangements

- For a private company to collect the body and carry out owner's wishes for burial, cremation in mass, or individual cremation with return of the ashes.
- For cremation with other bodies by the local authority.

If the body is left, do not immediately put it in the freezer. Owners often change their minds.

Owners can contact private companies

- Cremation, with or without return of the ashes.
- Burial in a pet cemetery, or a 'green burial' site.
- Acting as 'undertaker' and managing everything (home burials, memorial tree planting, even providing emotional support).

When utilizing facilities for disposal, there will be a cost. Prices vary enormously according to the locality, the sophistication of the services, the companies that offer them and the amount people actually **want** to spend.

Owners can bury animals themselves, or get help from family or friends

- Doing this together can be very healing for the whole family.
- If they own the ground home burial is very satisfying.
- The grave can be marked by stones, flowers, bushes or trees. Tending a grave gives owners a sense of still having some caring role for their animal.
- Some people bury dogs' bodies in wild areas (e.g. in the mountains) where they have walked together.

The bodies of small pets should also be respected and parents can help children to deal with this appropriately.

Other options

Preserving the animal's body in a way that it can be displayed, such as by taxidermy or freeze drying. This may seem strange to some, but if this is what is desired, it should be accepted.

Immediate care of the body

Whatever the option that has been decided, the body should always be treated with respect, and the owner's last view should be of the animal looking peaceful. **Never put a body in a bag when owners are around!** Even those who have no interest in a body after the animal has died are really upset if they see it put into a bin bag.

Home burial

Before clients take the body home for burial:

- Express the bladder and then wrap the body in a blanket or something supplied by the owner.
- Slip a plastic bag under the body in case of leakage.
- Some practices offer a range of commercially produced cardboard coffins.
- Warn the owner about the possibility of muscle twitching for a while.
- Advise the owner to have the animal in a position for burial before rigor mortis occurs.

When the animal is buried, advise the client to:

- Wrap the body in a favourite old coat or blanket.
- Place it in a heavy bag (do not seal in a plastic bag), a box or a coffin.
- Bury it about 3 feet deep if possible.
- Place some large stones on top, to make sure other animals do not interfere with it.

A problem with home burial arises if the owner moves house. The dilemma is whether to leave the remains, maybe to have them disturbed by the new owners, or to dig them up again and take them to the new home. Either way it can be difficult.

Cremation

Most crematoriums have a range of boxes or caskets for containing the ashes. The ashes (called 'cremains' in the US) become very significant, a final hurdle to deal with. Never leave a message on someone's answer phone that the ashes are ready for collection.

Uplifting the ashes:

- Some clients find that coming to the surgery to collect the ashes is a difficult task.
- If they cannot face it, they could get a friend to accompany them or call at the surgery instead of them.

- The practice may be willing to deliver.

What might a client do with the ashes?

- Scatter them around favourite places or walks.
- Scatter or bury them in the garden.
- Keep them in a chosen place, maybe buying a special jar or box.

No arrangements required
Some people may not want to even think about the body, either because they cannot bear to, or because once the animal is dead, they do not feel that the body matters anymore. In either case the attending or helping person should respect the owner's needs and beliefs. Be aware that they may change their mind.

Rituals
These are a matter of individual choice, and depend on whether dealing with the body or ashes. For children it is really important to celebrate the life and death in some way, and what's appropriate for them may be helpful for adults as well.

Post mortem
- If a post mortem is to be done, make sure the owner knows that a total necropsy will mean that the body should not be returned.
- If the owner wants a post mortem but still wants the body back, a cosmetic post mortem can be done, but they must understand that there will be limits to the information revealed.
- It might be that an owner cannot cope with the death because there are too many unanswered questions. Without a post mortem it is as if there is no closure. They need to know why it died.
- It may be important to determine the cause of death for the protection of other animals at home.
- When an animal has been ill and under treatment, a post mortem may provide some answers that may be helpful for the vet as well as the owner.
- Owners may feel that by allowing a post mortem, other animals may be helped ... that 'Tibby did not die in vain.'
- The owner should be prewarned that basic post mortems do not always reveal the answers.
- Where there are insurance claims, a post mortem may be required.

The final decision about post mortems is up to the owner. It may be quite all right for them, but on the other hand very upsetting.

People have said

- When the vet put Jason (my old Doberman) down, he was really kind, and though I was feeling bad, I was all right. Then he asked me to help put him in this black bin bag. I got really upset. I'll never forget that; it was as if he were rubbish; that was the worst part.
- I had not planned on leaving Tiggy's body, but it all happened so quickly, that I could not think straight. I had to run out. Now I really feel guilty that I did not bring her home to bury in the garden.
- I keep wondering why Sam died. I cannot stop thinking that it was my fault. I wish I had asked the vet to do a post mortem.
- I totally broke down when the voice on the answerphone said 'Your dog's ashes are ready for collection now'.
- My mum flushed my goldfish down the toilet before I could stop her.
- My dad helped me to bury my hamster in a little box in the garden.

HOME-BASED EUTHANASIA

This is an important issue for clients and should be considered as an option. Assume euthanasia decisions have been discussed and the owner has asked for it to be performed at home.

Benefit to the animal

- Dying in familiar surroundings with family near.
- Less psychological stress for nervous or fearful animals.
- Less physical hardship for animal which is ill, or distressed, in not having to be moved.

Benefits to the owner

- Avoids the emotionally disturbing last journey (guilt at taking animals to be killed).
- Safer for the owner not to have to drive.
- Privacy, not having to see anyone afterwards.
- The rest of the family can be there or not, without having to decide beforehand.
- The owner feels more in control of the situation.

- Owner feels that they have done the right thing, so they may not be so guilty.
- They will not associate the clinic with the animal's death.
- Easier for home burial, as the animal will not need transporting.

Benefits to the vet

- It seems more appropriate for the pet. Some vets feel more comfortable about it.
- There are no distractions (other clients, phone calls, reps, staff, etc.).
- It allows the vet to engage wholly with the client in their own environment.
- Home burial is facilitated, as there is no transporting of the body.
- The client does not develop a negative association with the practice.

Possible disadvantages of home euthanasia

- It takes up more of the vet's time.
- There is no back-up if things go wrong.
- Animals are apt to be more assertive (aggressive) in their own territory.
- The light is often poor.
- The vet may have to transport heavy dogs back to the surgery.

Find out
- If the animal is likely to be difficult (check records).
- Who wants to be present.
- The preferred method of dealing with the body.

Action
- Always bring an assistant.
- Ensure all necessary routine equipment is included, making provision for emergencies. Have appropriate restraint equipment available in car (collar, lead, muzzle, cat restraint basket); head torch if lighting is very poor; old blanket for carrying out animal; plastic sheet to slip under body; roll of paper towel for mess.
- If a heavy dog's body is to be taken back to the surgery, back the car into a good position for ease of loading the body. This makes leaving less traumatic for the owner to witness.

- Make sure the animal is contained in a room where it can be retrieved easily, thus preventing awkward catching problems, especially with cats.
- Decide with the owner where it should be done. *Outside*: make sure the animal cannot run off; aesthetically more pleasant, animal often more relaxed; no room associated with memories; cleaner if animal defecates and urinates. *Inside*: kitchen floor usually easier to clean up than others. If carpeted room, best if animal can rest on its blanket; if none, bring one from the car. If animal is settled in a place, do it there if possible.
- Carry out routines as described in 'Client-present euthanasia'.
- Make the animal look comfortable and attend to the owner.
- Afterwards, if it seems appropriate, stay with the owner for a few minutes.
- The owner will indicate if they want to talk or to be left alone.
- Before leaving, say something reassuring, comforting and acknowledging the loss (whatever seems right at the time).
- Carry out the body wrapped in a blanket or an old coat supplied by the owner (something they can still do for the animal). For a big dog use a blanket as a stretcher.
- Do not use a plastic bag except as a sheet to slip under the body.
- If there is to be a home burial, offer to help carry a large animal outside or suggest something to be placed under the body indoors. Warn about possible tremors and rigor mortis.
- Settle body in a good looking comfortable position wrapped in a favourite old coat or blanket. Leaving the head out is more acceptable.

Comment

Memories are so important. Take great care to prevent trouble. The potential for things to go wrong is greater in home euthanasia and if this should happen, the owner may be left with a permanent painful recollection of what happened in that room in the house. Every detail must be meticulously considered, in order that the memories should be of the animal slipping away peacefully in its own home.

If euthanasias are in the veterinary surgery, some clients cannot bear to return there with another animal, even though everything had gone perfectly and they had been very grateful to the vet. This is a strong argument for home euthanasia.

A vet writes:

Home euthanasia will always stand out as some of the most rewarding and memorable moments of my work. If done well, it can be deeply rewarding and warrant the extra time and trouble it involves. I think owners are always extremely grateful for the effort.

Sir Chris Bonnington writes:

Most of our animals have lived to a good old age, but there comes a time when because of various ailments their quality of life is so poor that it is kinder to have them put down. Our local vet has always been really good and has been happy to come out to our home to give that fatal injection. He has done it in a way that our dog or cat has hardly known what was happening. They did not have to go through the trauma of being taken to the vet; it is the difference in human terms of dying at home surrounded by your friends and family instead of in the impersonal, clinical environment of a hospital.

EUTHANASIA OF HORSES

Although equines are longer lived than smaller companion animals, they frequently have had changes in ownership and are sold on to other owners. Relationships with horses are not always expected to continue indefinitely as with other companion animals. Even so, when they die it is very distressing for most owners as it involves parting with a good friend as well as a working animal. It may be, especially with some children, that the animal has occupied most of their leisure time as well as providing a means for social activities with other horse or pony owners.

Reasons for euthanasia

Healthy animals
Unlike small animals, healthy horses are not usually euthanased.

- If they do not perform well they can be sold on, or sold for the meat market. (Most owners with a close attachment to their horses would not consider selling them for meat.)
- If they have a dangerous behaviour problem they may be slaughtered at an abattoir licensed for horses (providing they have not received medication).

Injured, sick or ageing animals

Injury

- Animals critically injured in accidents may have to be immediately euthanased.
- Decisions have to be made quickly, often by distraught owners who may themselves be injured.
- This may happen at a public event, and is harrowing for everyone.

Economics and insurance cover may be critical factors in decisions involving injuries which may not be life threatening, but present a poor outlook for future performance.

Illness

Animals which are acutely or chronically ill, unable to work, or are not treatable on economic or humane grounds may be euthanased. The same process of decision making should be followed as for other companion animals, except that these are dual purpose animals, and their function is also a consideration. Economics and insurance are important factors.

Ageing

Elderly animals retired from work often become neglected, living alone in fields with only their basic needs met. Owners feel that they should still keep them but they may not be aware how miserable their lives might become. Being social animals, used to lots of care and attention, they at least need good feeding and other equine company. If aged animals cannot be provided with good care and attention, the humane alternatives are to re-home them with a rescue or to have them euthanased.

Pre-euthanasia discussion

This will be as for small animals. This is the time for the vet to be caring and sensitive to the owner's feelings. However, the options are not the same for owner participation and this will have to be made very clear. There should not be arguments at the death.

Owners must not be allowed to hold the horse or try to comfort it during the death. The death may be distressing to witnesses and they could be severely injured or killed if the horse fell on them.

The procedure

- The potential dangers are great and the vet needs to take charge of the situation with firmness.
- If it is an emergency in a public place, the vet should send every-one away, even if it means getting incredibly bossy.
- Even the owners should be encouraged to say their goodbyes and then leave.
- Whatever the method of killing, it is vital to have a good handler on the head, to steady the animal and to ensure it falls the right way. (If not managed, the horse will pitch forward).
- Whatever the method of killing, it is best to sedate the animal first.

Chemical death

- The use of an intravenous cannula taped in before the main injection prevents the needle popping out as the animal falls. Make sure the horse falls with the line uppermost.
- Some products act quicker than others. With the slower ones you may have to wait a long time before the heart finally stops beating.
- A chemical death is quiet and fairly peaceful, but the meat cannot be used.

Shooting

- Is quick, but potentially dangerous and requires a licensed expert.
- Knackers can be called in and are usually very humane and efficient. They relieve the vet of a worrying job. They can remove the body immediately.
- In some areas, people from hunt kennels will come and do the job, and remove the body.
- Some owners do not like shooting as it seems violent; they hear the shot and they may think the other horses will be upset.

The body

Ask the owners beforehand if they would like a switch of hair to keep.

- Contact the knackers and tell them when you will be performing the euthanasia. They will arrange to come within a few minutes of the death.

- If the owners want to see their animal after a chemical death, let them come and say goodbye.
- If there has been a shooting, it is very distressing for them to see the body.
- Cover the body with a rug or tarpaulin.
- Make sure that sensitive owners, especially children, do not stay to see the animal picked up.
- Their last image should be as normal as possible, certainly not of an animal being winched onto a lorry, either bound for local hunt kennels or the knackers yard.

Even when owners pay vast amounts for burial or cremation, the transportation is the same distressing process.

Comment

The death, transportation and the final destination of the body are all potentially very distressing for a caring owner. Vets should be aware of and acknowledge the emotional hardship for many owners, especially for the children. There is traditionally little understanding or support for sorrowing owners.

NOTES

Challenging or special situations

1

Helping clients through emotional difficulties

GUILTY CLIENTS

Feelings of guilt are almost inevitable following a significant human bereavement, and concern a lifetime of unfinished business and regrets for past actions or inactions. Guilt following an animal death centres mostly on the circumstances leading up to the death, the manner of death and the period afterwards, and is especially prevalent when euthanasia decisions have been made.

Guilt can be damaging to client's well-being and block their progress through grief. Excessive guilt causes such pain and distress that it can lead to unresolved, even pathological, grieving.

What do clients feel guilty about?

The most common source of guilt can be anticipated. Some guilt is completely inappropriate in that a person may assume responsibility for something that they could have had no influence over (e.g. an animal developing cancer).

They may even feel guilty about showing emotions, for 'breaking down' in the surgery.

People say they feel guilty because:

- They did not really understand the situation before making decisions.
- They had not been encouraged to ask questions.
- They feel they should have asked for another opinion or changed vets.
- They feel that maybe they should have delayed longer before deciding on euthanasia.
- They feel that maybe they left it too long and the animal may have been suffering.
- The animal was frightened at the surgery; they should have insisted on a home euthanasia.
- They could not endure staying with the animal at the death.

- They did not go in afterwards and say goodbye (and they wonder if it really did die).
- They should not have left the body with the vet.
- They did not handle things right and the children were upset with them.
- They made the 'wrong choice' about how the body was disposed of (i.e. burial or cremation).
- Children often feel guilty for and responsible about decisions made by parents.

The list goes on – it seems that no matter what people do, they manage to feel guilty. Some of these reasons reflect a general lack of confidence in the vet, many seem to be the direct result of poor communication and some are caused by poor or uninformed planning

Vets, being aware of the potential power of guilt, can try to ensure understanding, encourage clients to ask questions and to consider all the options **before** making final decisions.

After an animal's death, especially when by euthanasia, if the client says 'I feel so guilty', acknowledge their feelings and then help them explore the source of guilt. It is not so helpful just to tell them they should not feel that way.

When genuine mistakes are made, or inattention leads to misfortune, the guilt is understandable and reasonable. The situation needs to be faced and worked through, the feelings acknowledged, not brushed off or minimized. Let them know, however, that it is normal to feel the way they do, at the same time as reassuring them that they had loved their animal and done their best for him/her.

> *Carrying a load of guilt is like carrying a rucksack full of stones. If you want, or need, to carry it, you can; or you could take out a few stones and lighten it a bit, or you could even empty the whole lot and travel free. It is completely up to the person, but sometimes it is very hard to let the guilt go.*

ANGRY CLIENTS

Anger is a basic reaction to losing something that is valued. Nevertheless when a loved animal has been helped into peaceful death, the owner may feel no anger at all, only sadness and even gratitude for the care taken and kindness shown.

Remember that the potential for an angry response is always there.

In the state of heightened awareness experienced at the time of death, the owner is acutely sensitive to everything that happens, good or bad. It does not take much to mobilize that anger.

To avoid anger

Have a good understanding of how clients experience animal death. **All the staff should make great efforts to be kind and caring throughout the encounter, avoiding any detrimental or careless words or actions.**

How to help angry clients

The way the client's anger is handled at this time is critical to their acceptance of the death and their progress towards resolution.

- If a client is very angry, do not immediately get defensive or feel victimized.
- If you are anxious or doubtful about decisions made, and avoid eye contact, the client will pick that up.
- Keep calm and make sure you have all the facts; then ask the client to join you in a place where you can sit down together and talk privately. This gives you an appearance of control and gives the client a chance to cool down.
- Acknowledging their anger, demonstrate that you are interested in hearing about their complaints.
- Let them blow off steam, but warn them if you are reaching your limits.
- If there has been an obvious reason for a client's anger, maybe a grossly careless attitude or a genuine mistake made, it should be faced in an honest and sensitive way. Their emotions can be acknowledged without taking over the responsibility for them. Try to find some basis for agreement and compromise.
- After a death, people in shock may be searching for a meaning, an understanding of what happened.
- Angry clients need recognition of their feelings and may genuinely want some answers to questions that are troubling them.
- Vets should realise that there are often no answers, but should show a willingness to hear the questions.

Anger that is allowed expression usually dispels itself as long as you have the tolerance, patience and courage to see it through. Anger that is blocked, not acknowledged and not allowed expression often

escalates, until people feel the need to act on it, maybe by making a formal complaint or starting a court action.
  Do not:

- Make outright admissions of error, but if possible demonstrate flexibility. 'I can see your point'. Avoid following on with '**but**', which just negates what has been said
- Get angry back at them.
- Argue or put them off with defensive excuses, so that they are left feeling unacknowledged and powerless. This often results in people making complaints in order to get some sort of satisfaction.

If a client will not calm down and talk rationally, you could say, in a soft firm voice, that you would like to discuss this but it is impossible when they are so angry and ask them to leave just now.

If you are concerned that a client is likely to be dangerously out of control, make sure that you have someone else around.

Personal response to anger in general

Be aware of your own response to anger. Think of occasions when you have had angry clients. Ask yourself, 'How do I respond when people are angry at me? Do I get angry as well? Do I get fearful and anxious? How does it affect my well-being afterwards? Do I feel misunderstood and less confident?'.

If you have difficulty coping with anger in yourself or from others, it may be that a few hours spent at an anger workshop or communication skills training course may be well worth the time and effort.

A vet writes:

A dog was euthanased because of renal failure. Her owner arrived at the surgery a few days later, very angry at the incompetence of the practice vets and considering 'further action'. I was sick with the flu, but ushered him into my office. For 40 minutes he raged on. I was too ill to argue against his unjust tirade, and just let it crash over me. Gradually his aggression lessened, giving way to sadness and tears. Then he said he felt much better, and realized that I was busy and should get back to my work. I told him that he'd had his say and now I'd have mine. He anticipated my rage, but I told him that I could understand his reactions, and acknowledged his sadness at losing Trixie. I spoke a bit about the emotions that accompany pet loss. We spoke of Trixie and what she had meant to him. He explained that she had been instrumental in rebuilding his confidence following a stroke many years before. He was surprised and relieved by my understanding. He left as one of our most grateful clients. If I had not been ill, I would have countered his unfounded claims and not allowed him to vent his feelings. I now have more confidence in speaking with angry clients, encouraging them to get things off their chest, and carefully listening to what they say.'

CLIENTS WHO TALK ABOUT 'JUST WANTING TO DIE'

Do not panic! **Remain calm and confident, and let them know you've heard what they are saying. You may say something like 'It sounds as if life does not seem worth living for you just now' or 'I guess life will seem pretty empty for you without Jody'. Most people who say they want to die are not actually suicidal; they just want to express how bad it is or how desolate they are feeling.**

Case report

An old Alsatian had just been euthanased. His distraught elderly owner, lying on the floor holding the body in his arms, sobbed and he said he just wanted to be dead too. The attending vet did not know what to do, but just let him lie there for a while, then put a hand on his shoulder and said something about how much he had loved his dog. The nurse brought him a cup of tea and sat with him, just staying with whatever he said. When he left they checked that he was OK to go home on his own. They sent him a note that day. He wrote in to say how grateful he was for their care.

- Do not try to make people 'feel better by looking at the sunny side', what they really need at that moment is for you to understand how bad it is for them.
- It is crucial that you do not rush them out. They must have some time to recover before facing the world.
- If you really think they are serious about suicide and they tell you they are really going to do it, do not be scared to talk about it.
- If you know they have other animals you might ask about who would look after them.

Comment
A vet writes:

*I find the word **validation** useful in describing one of the chief tasks of the veterinary team with regard to pet owners' responses to their* *pets. I like to think of my practice as being the one place where they have the freedom to be totally open and accepted with respect to their relationship with their pet. By validating their experience, particularly of grief, we can do a lot to assure them that they are not alone, unusual or insane.*

How can you get further help for a troubled client?

- When you feel that the situation is really serious, you might want to consult with a colleague. Be prepared to suggest contacting the Samaritans (24 hours a day) or counsellors affiliated with a medical practice. Private counselling may be beyond the client's resources.
- Although it is best that clients stay in control of their situation themselves, it may be that a client will ask you to contact their GP for them, fearing that the doctor might take grieving over an animal death as a *bona fide* reason for seeking counselling.
- In less critical situations there are other sources of help such as SCAS/Blue Cross Befrienders service or maybe local groups or individuals (who have passed your personal scrutiny).
- The practice should keep a list of contact numbers.

How should you approach this? Though it is not your responsibility to make arrangements, or to be at all directive, you can help them decide whether or not they need help from others. You might ask them if they have anything in mind, and follow on from what they lead with. You could say something like, 'This may not be appropriate, but we have a leaflet about a service that you may want to contact. It is entirely up to you what you do with it.'.

How do vets cope?

The effectiveness of vets in coping with these very traumatic experiences will be based on the vets' ability to look after themselves.

A vet states:

Our job provides enormous emotional rewards. It strikes me that the price we must pay for this return is to engage with the client/pet and become to some degree involved and affected by the process. There can be no free lunch. The skill comes in being able to avoid becoming totally immersed in the personal drama of each situation.

Out of your depth

As vets and nurses involved with emotional clients you might find yourself getting drawn into situations for which you have neither the time or the necessary skills.

You need to establish boundaries.

- **Professional boundaries** are defined by your job and responsibilities. As veterinary staff you have loyalty and responsibility to the practice as well as to the clients, and should avoid getting embroiled in issues which do not involve the animals.
- **Personal boundaries** very much depend on what you feel comfortable with and that in turn may be influenced by your own emotional experience. Unresolved issues may interfere with your ability to be wholly with the client's situation. Those who have had recent major losses are usually advised to take time out before dealing with the grief of others.

In all instances, a balance must be maintained between too much and too little personal involvement. Too much involvement, especially when dealing with very needy clients, may lead to stress and burn out for you, and some over-dependent clients. This would not be beneficial for either of you. Too little involvement and a distancing approach may deprive you of the rewarding aspects of your work, and may leave clients feeling that no one really cares and that neither they nor their animals have been valued.

It is a recurrent problem for those in the 'helping professions' that in order to function effectively, to enjoy being a good doctor, nurse (or vet) they must allow themselves to approach, and to a degree, share the distress of those they are attempting to help.

(Dr Colin Murray Parkes)

2

Disabled clients

Many people with disabilities have companion animals. They may be pets or assistance animals, usually dogs, which have been trained to help them with their particular difficulty.

Veterinary practices should be equipped to offer effective and satisfactory service to all of their clients. The Disability Discrimination Act 1995 provides that 'businesses open to the public must make reasonable adjustments to accommodate disabled people'.

A recent survey showed that one in six of the population of the UK have some degree of disability. The vast majority (about 94%) of these people have become disabled during their lifetime, in other words were not born disabled, and have been fully integrated in society. The implication of this for all of us who are not at the moment disabled is that we might consider ourselves to be 'temporarily able bodied'. Chances are that, if we live long enough, we will at some point in our lives become disabled in some respect. It is useful to remember this if we find ourselves becoming patronising in our relationships with disabled clients. In fact it would be highly beneficial for vets or their staff to attend a course on Disability Equality Awareness Training. If a disabled client is accompanied by a non-disabled person, direct your communication and attention to the client, not to their companion. As for all clients, check for understanding and encourage questions. Avoid treating clients in a patronising manner.

BLIND AND VISUALLY IMPAIRED CLIENTS

- Introduce yourself and any attending staff. Speak to the client as much as possible.
- Use your normal voice in tone and volume. Just because they are blind does not mean they are deaf.

- Give a running commentary while assessing the animal, explaining what examinations you are carrying out and what you are finding.
- Discuss the treatment and describe in detail what you are doing or propose to do.
- When deciding on medications, if there is an option of liquid or pills, ask the client's preference.
- Dispense them in containers which are easily identifiable by shape or size, or you can mark them distinctively with tape or rubber bands.
- If liquid medication is used, have a way of measuring dosages, maybe with a notched syringe.
- Demonstrate and then watch the client practise giving medication (using water or bread pellets).
- Ensure that the client understands and feels confident administering treatment.
- Give an opportunity to ask questions and offer to write down instructions. If the client is anxious, it can be difficult to take everything in and there may be someone at home to help.
- If you are performing euthanasia, describe in detail every move you are making and what the animal might be experiencing.

DEAF AND HEARING-IMPAIRED CLIENTS

- Show the client what you are doing.
- Always face the client when talking, never talk while turning your face away.
- Determine what communication style is used, whether lip reading or signing.
- If an interpreter is being used, direct your statements to the client, not the interpreter.
- Write down details of the diagnosis and instructions for treatment.
- Find out from a telephone company (BT) about using the 'Type Talk' service.
- Encourage a member of staff to attend a class teaching signing. This is appreciated by deaf clients. Word gets around and deaf owners are more likely to choose your practice.

Physically disabled clients

- Be flexible with appointments, since many disabled people rely on others for transport.
- Ensure that clients are enabled to access your premises and that facilities are provided.
- If this is temporarily not possible to arrange, be prepared to make home visits.
- When talking to a client, sit level with the client's chair.
- If a client is in a wheel chair, treat the animal on a low table if possible or on the floor.
- Ask the client about his/her ability to give medication or to carry out tasks associated with treatments, such as cleaning out ears.
- Work out a regime of treatment that will accommodate the client's physical abilities
- Give a 'hands on' demonstration, then ask the client to practise it.
- Always deal with the disabled person directly, not with anyone accompanying them.
- If an animal is being euthanased, it is important that the procedure is carried out at a level to enable the owner to hold the animal.

Disabled clients with assistance animals

There are several charity-based organisations involved in the training and supplying of assistance dogs to disabled people. These include The Guide Dogs for the Blind Association (GDBA), Hearing Dogs for Deaf People (HDFD), Dogs for the Disabled (DFD), Canine Partners for Independence (CPI) and 'Support Dogs'.

- Professionally trained assistance dogs can be recognized by the special harnesses or identifying jackets.
- Most organizations that provide and train the dogs, provide insurance cover for veterinary costs or meet the costs from their own funds.
- Guide dog owners are the legal owners of their dogs. (On qualifying they purchase their dog for a nominal sum. From then on the owner has ultimate legal responsibility for the dog's actions and for any costs incurred. GDBA does, however, meet all the feeding and veterinary costs.)

Some other organizations (CPI) retain ownership and may recall a dog if it is no longer able to work due to illness, age or other problems, or if the partnership is not successful for any reason. Although the client may not be the legal owner, 'owner' is still used in the text here. 'Support Dogs' are usually pet dogs belonging to a person with a disability but trained by 'Support Dogs' to perform required tasks.

An assistance dog may almost seem to become a 'part' of the person. The relationship is qualitatively different from that with a pet dog, because of the inter-dependency that takes place. The dog develops a sense of responsibility and nurture towards the person, and the person relies upon the dog for increased independence, as well as constant companionship.

All the information about disabled pet owners applies here. There are some important differences, however.

- In cases where the dog is the property of the providing organization (as in CPI), that organization will be involved as well as the clients, when veterinary care is required. The GDBA view is that owners should remain in control of what happens to their dog, but that GDBA will provide as much care/support/back-up as required (including their own vet to carry out an operation if necessary with aftercare performed by the staff). They do insist on being kept informed – usually after the event but preferably before if a non-urgent operation is necessary.
- The owners have been selected, screened and trained to take the very best care of their animals, and may be more observant than others of any change that might indicate a problem.
- The animals provide assistance, which the owners have come to depend upon, so there is a potential need for house calls if the dog is ill.
- While ensuring the very best veterinary care available, if there are several options, the treatment that is least likely to affect the working partnership should be employed.
- The dog should only be admitted if it is really necessary. Inform the owner if you think the treatment will affect the dog's physical or mental abilities.
- They should also be warned if there might be changes in the dog's usual functions, such as needing to urinate or defecate more frequently.

Do not make assumptions about an owner's difficulty, just because you cannot perceive any.

- Some owners have 'hidden' disabilities and their dogs are specially trained to help them, e.g. seizure alert dogs and support dogs for unsteady walkers.

- When in doubt, ask: 'Can you tell me what you think I need to know about your condition?'.
- Ask the client about the role of the animal and the tasks it does.
- Ask (do not make assumptions) about who takes care of or exercises the dog.
- Even severely disabled clients frequently develop sophisticated ways of coping with their environment to maintain a high degree of functional independence.

Handling and dealing with assistance animals

- Ideally introduce the dog to the surgery at an initial visit before any treatment is required.
- Approach the animal in a gentle fashion.
- Ask what commands the dog will respond to before resorting to physical restraint, e.g. lying down rather than being forced down.
- Some assistance dogs are very sensitive to an approach by a stranger and may be intimidated by a perceived threat behaviour, which can include direct eye contact, standing or leaning over the dog, or staring it in the face.
- They may be overwhelmed by rough handling, even though playful, and probably because of this, some trainers think that some male vets are more intimidating than female vets.
- Many guide dogs are temperamentally sensitive but because of their upbringing and training are not expected to be easily intimidated.

Simple behaviours used to calm dogs in the surgery
- Not making direct eye contact.
- Standing alongside rather than in front of the dog, facing in the same direction as the dog.
- Talking to the owner while crouching or kneeling beside the dog.
- Yawning and 'softening' the facial expression by smiling.
- Blinking when looking at the dog.
- Telling jokes and laughing with the owner.
- A dog may be encouraged to jump on the scales, or get up on to a table, through playful persuasion by the owner using a toy or squeaker.

Seriously ill animals
When assistance animals become seriously ill the following points should be noted:

- The organisation which has trained and supplied the dogs maintains an interest in them, and responsibility towards both the animals and the owners.
- GDBA has access to a wide variety of leading consultants at various veterinary schools. In many cases they can arrange early appointments and have preferred specialists for referral, so if a guide dog needs a referral, contact GDBA.
- If the providing organization owns the dog, any possibility of euthanasia must be discussed with the organization, as well as with the client. This may be difficult in an emergency, and the vet taking on the health care of the dog should be informed of the official procedure if this should occur.
- GDBA does not require advance notice of euthanasia, or signed consent, but should be informed where possible in order to provide support.
- If euthanasia is being considered as an option, the client should be given time if possible to adjust to the situation. This is important not only because of the emotional impact, but because of the practical aspects of re-arranging their lifestyle to cope without a dog, including extra care assistants and emergency arrangements where necessary.
- If possible, euthanasia should take place in the owner's home.
- If the death/euthanasia is sudden and unexpected, the owner may need help getting home. **All the information given for carrying out euthanasia that causes owners the minimum of distress pertains particularly to the euthanasia of an assistance dog. The owners should be offered a pre-euthanasia discussion. This will help them think clearly about options (e.g. cremation or burial).**
- If the cause of death is not known and the dog is relatively young, the GDBA might request a post mortem but only with the consent of the owner. The impact of this death on the life and well-being of the owner may be considerable.
- The person is suddenly deprived not only of a valued partner, but also of the independent lifestyle and perceived social acceptability that the assistance dog had contributed.
- The resulting deprivation of independence creates a profound sense of loss, the assistance animal having helped to remove many of the barriers to disabled people that exist in society.
- In some cases, the initial feelings of loss associated with the disability might be reactivated.
- If the dog was still working, there may be some delay before a new dog can be provided.

- The replacement with a new dog may not be as successful as the original partnership.
- Barriers to new relationships may be due to unresolved grief for the animal that has died.
- Some organizations have bereavement counsellors as part of the support personnel available to their graduates. Some will pay for cremation (GDBA).
- GDBA centres have gardens of remembrance, where ashes can be scattered and plaques placed in memory of the guide dog.
- If your client is greatly distressed, you should be able to supply information about support groups as well as the names of local *bona fide* counsellors, especially those that specialise in grief work. (You should personally check out any person that you are recommending. Some 'pet bereavement counsellors' may have had little or no counselling education.)

3

Clients from different cultures or ethnic backgrounds

LANGUAGE DIFFICULTIES

Ease of communication may be influenced by how integrated the client is into western culture. Some immigrant populations live in a close community and if the older people are not using English very much, they might have difficulty with discussions about a sick pet's illness or options for treatment. It is always a good idea to suggest that they are accompanied by a younger family member.

RELIGIOUS OR CULTURAL INFLUENCES

In the west we accept that euthanasia to end the suffering of our animals is a humane and acceptable action.

- Some clients are unable to accept euthanasia on religious/cultural grounds.
- When faced with such a situation in which an animal is in a terminal condition and clearly suffering it is best not to force the issue. Insisting that the only option is euthanasia may create an atmosphere of antagonism. Try to explain your concerns.
- Ensure that you have allowed ample time to discuss the situation.
- Make sure someone is present to act as a translator in order to avoid misunderstandings.
- If the animal's condition is not immediately critical, it may be best, after a full discussion, to send it home with some palliative care and suggest the owner returns after they have had a chance to discuss things in private.
- In some circumstances, suggest they speak with a priest of their own religion as sometimes these matters are not quite as clear cut as the client believes them to be.

- A family conference, either at home or in the clinic, tends to be successful because of the influence of the younger family members, although it is important for the vet to make a direct contact with the head of the family.
- Occasionally it may be necessary to make a follow-up phone call to ensure the pet is coming back or receiving appropriate care.

It may be easy to assume that because of different customs and body language, because the animals are not spoken to so much and are often kept outside, members of the Asian community are less caring. However, that is misleading, for animals are often considered to be part of the family and well loved.

A sense of dignity may discourage emotional involvement with people outside of the family but the support within the family is strong.

- When an animal is euthanased, often a large group of family members will accompany the pet to say goodbye and after the death may require time to console each other. This can result in the room being out of use for some time.
- The body is usually taken away for burial. If possible, try to arrange that another exit from the surgery is available.
- Very occasionally, euthanasia will not be permitted. It is important to maintain adequate client relationships so that the pet is provided with palliative care.
- It is a difficult ethical situation and you may want guidance from the RCVS.

Sometimes clients will appear to be more concerned with the economic loss associated with their pet's condition, than an emotional involvement with the animal. In these circumstances, a euthanasia decision is fairly straightforward and little emotion is shown. However, it is not a vet's role to make a judgement about whether a person or family is grieving or not. Cultural differences may influence both expressions and perceptions. In all cases maintain a caring attitude and stay respectful of your client's autonomy.

4
Clients who wish referral to complementary medicine

The public in general is beginning to have an interest in complementary medicine and many people use these approaches in dealing with their health problems. It is not surprising that pet owners may specifically request access to natural medicine for their animals. A request for information about, or a referral for, such therapies does not normally indicate that a client wishes to abandon conventional medicine, or leave their usual practice. It does mean that the client wishes to explore another route in addition to conventional veterinary practice, i.e. complementary rather than alternative medicine.

- If this is the case it is far better to refer a client to a veterinary colleague, with the advantage of a background in conventional medicine, rather than risking the client going to a 'lay' homeopath, herbalist, etc.
- If vets are worried about the animal's safety, they can feel reassured that natural medicine will not adversely interact with any conventional medicine.
- If they are concerned because they 'do not believe in it' they can be honest with the client about that while still giving them the autonomy to do what they want.
- Clients should not have to feel guilty or be afraid of a vet's reactions, especially if their own doctor is comfortable with complementary approaches to their personal health.
- Vets who co-operate with clients in this area find that the clients have great loyalty to them because of their understanding and willingness to respect their clients' choices.

Many vets who practise conventional medicine have started to branch out and may have certain clinics just for patients who prefer to use complementary methods as well.

NOTES

Subjects owners may want information about

1

Children and pet loss

For many of us the death of a childhood pet was our first experience of major loss. The details surrounding the death and the memory of our emotions at that time often remain vivid long after the memory of other early losses has faded.

If a person wants to help a child who is losing or has lost a pet, it is useful to consider several things which may affect the way children experience loss and express grief.

- The age, and the individual development and personal experience of the child.
- The nature and strength of the attachment to and relationship with the animal.
- The circumstances of the loss or death and the child's involvement.
- The child's relationship with parents or significant adults.
- The sensitivity and skill of significant adults in understanding and providing support.
- Presence of other animals.

AGE AND COGNITIVE DEVELOPMENT OF CHILDREN

To a certain extent these go together, but there is great individual variation and some children mature a lot faster than others.

- Very young children (up to 2 years of age) have no concept of death, but may miss the presence of an animal and will be aware of tensions in the family if others are grieving. If so they may become clingy and whining, needing reassurance.
- As they approach school age, children are developing quickly and are very curious about the world around them. They are fascinated by dead butterflies and other small creatures, often bringing them to their parents and asking questions. Having played

games where they are shot dead and jump up again, and seen cartoons where indestructible animals revive immediately after terrible traumas, they have difficulty with the concept of death as being permanent.

- Parents who take advantage of opportunities to talk about death will be helping prepare their children for when or if a pet should die. If that should happen, the child may need to be told patiently over and over again that the pet is dead and will not be coming back. Children's grief may show in different ways; they may regress and need lots of reassurance, or they may be difficult, or over-anxious, or weepy. Since their attention span is short, they may suddenly seem to forget and start playing, then later get upset again.
- With encouragement and comfort, young children may work through grief quite quickly.
- Around their early school years, children are into magical thinking. Death may appear to be some evil being, which can be controlled by 'heroes'. If they themselves are the 'heroes', they may feel somehow responsible that they had not prevented a death or they may feel the death was their fault, that it was a punishment for their bad thoughts or deeds. In fact guilty children may behave badly, so that they receive the 'deserved' punishment. At this time they are gradually becoming aware that death is permanent, but hoping that it maybe does not happen to everyone.
- Children of all ages may worry about the dead pet being lonely or cold in its grave, even though they know it is dead. Even some adults can have sensations of such thoughts
- From 9 years of age, most children have become aware of the biological finality of death. They may be curious about what happens to bodies or what happens in post mortems, and they need honest and direct answers. They may worry a lot about the death of people they love. They may worry that people they love might die and need reassurance, if they ask. This is an important time to have 'good talks' about life and death.
- Adolescence is a time of high emotions and confusion. Adolescents may be less willing to share feelings or talk to parents about real issues. In fact they may feel closer to an animal than to their family; it may be the only one they feel totally relaxed with, that they can cuddle or confide in. The death of such a pet at that time of transition can be devastating. Adolescents, especially boys who are trying to prove their manhood, may be distressed and embarrassed by the strength of their grief. They may want to be treated as an adult and yet have the needs of a really hurt

child. Basically they should be given every opportunity to talk and share their feelings, without putting on them any expectations as to how they should be.

- Whatever the age of the child, it is important to remember that though they may be experiencing grief as much as an adult, they may express it in different ways.

Adults should NOT assume things about the way a child is feeling, without checking it out with the child. They may be resentful, uncooperative, sulky, unable to concentrate at school and parents might not recognize that grief could be the source of these behaviours.

> ... the suggestion often to emerge in families that because a child did not express grief in the manner of adults, he did not grieve or care.
>
> (Mgt Torrie)

THE RELATIONSHIP THAT HAS BEEN LOST

Encouraging the child to talk about the animal will help in the understanding of what impact the loss may have. Some children are quite casual and not deeply involved with their pet; some may even be a bit relieved that they do not have to look after it any more. However, most children are fond of their pets, and for some, their animals have been really important and special in their lives.

Things children have mentioned as making an animal special:

- She was my first pet.
- It is the first time anything depended on me.
- I rescued it from a horrible cage in a pet shop.
- It was always there through my childhood.
- I had no sister or brother so he was like my brother.
- She was my best pal.
- She was the only one who understood when I was upset.
- I could tell him all my troubles, and he never got mad at me.

An animal may have been an important part of a child's social life

- He was the best pony in the world. We were in the games team together. I do not have him to ride or look after, and I cannot be in the team anymore.
- The other children used to come over because they liked to play with my dog.

An animal may be a link with a loved person that has left or died.

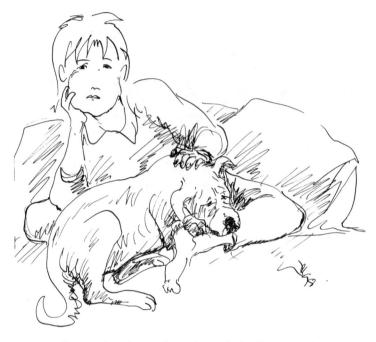

'She was the only one who understood when I was upset.'

- He was my uncle's dog, he was all we had left of my uncle and now he's gone too.

   Sometimes an animal has represented stability in times of transition or traumas:

- He got me through my exams.
- He was the only thing I could count on when my parents split up.
- We moved house and I had to leave all my friends. I only had my dog to play with.
- When I was ill and had to stay in bed a lot, my cat kept me company and never left me.

CIRCUMSTANCES OF LOSS OR DEATH AND THE CHILD'S ROLE

- When the death of an animal is anticipated, through illness or growing disability, the way it is handled makes a great difference to the children.

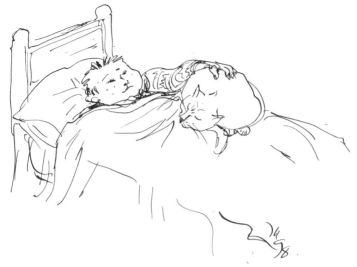

'When I was ill and had to stay in bed a lot, my cat kept me company and never left me.'

- If an animal is very ill, the parents might encourage children to spend time alone with it and comfort it. For older children, getting involved in the care of the animal gives them an insight into the gravity of the illness.
- This is an opportunity to answer questions and prepare them for the approaching death.
- Do not overload them with a lot of details; just answer simply, respecting their safety 'cut-off point'.
- Ensure that children do not get the idea that all illness leads to death.
- They should be told ill people usually get better, but sometimes bodies wear out or are so damaged that they cannot be fixed.

When there are decisions to be made about euthanasia, if it is possible children should be included and given time to voice their fears and ask questions.

Some children want to help comfort the animal while it is dying. This may be appropriate if everything is straightforward and the vet agrees. They should be told what they should do, what will be happening and what the animal will feel.

If they do not stay, they should at least be able to spend a few minutes saying goodbye before and after the death, if they want to.

- It is always very difficult when a death has been sudden, with everyone unprepared and not even able to say goodbye.
- If the body has been damaged, it is best to cover the injured parts, making it look as comfortable as possible; children should not be left with dreadful last images.
- Children may be shocked, disbelieving and horrified, feeling responsible, guilty and angry, as well as distressed and crying.
- They need to be assured that it was not their fault, to have their feelings acknowledged, and be comforted in their grief.

CASE STUDY – CHILD'S PERCEPTIONS

A distraught mother phoned her vet for advice. A week previously, the old ailing family dog had become extremely ill while the son was at school. The father took the dog to the vet surgery, where it was euthanased. Being very upset the father just wanted to get away quickly and left the body at the vet's. The unsuspecting 10-year-old son came home from school to find his dog had gone. His parents tried to tell him what happened, but he started shouting and screaming calling his dad a murderer.

Since then, the mother told the vet, the boy had been angry and then very morose, not eating much and just staying in his room. When his mother finally got him to talk he said he was angry at his dad and the vet, but he also felt it was his fault, that God was punishing him for being bad.

The vet offered to speak to the boy and came to the house to do so. After listening to the boy's perceptions, the vet explained about the dog's illness and how much it was suffering, so they had helped it to die peacefully. She answered his questions honestly and managed to convince him that no-one was to blame.

A month later the boy came to the surgery with a new puppy and seemed to be happy again.

RITUALS AND RITES OF PASSAGE

If the body is available, then some sort of rites of passage may be helpful for grieving children, as a way of saying the last goodbye.

Burial

- If burial is possible, then children can be encouraged to take part, maybe helping in choosing a spot, even doing some digging, putting flowers on the body, throwing in earth.

- Children may want some sort of saying goodbye ceremony, depending on their beliefs.
- They can decide on decorations for the grave, maybe marking the spot with stones or shells.
- Finding a grave stone; some children will make efforts to find just the right grave stone, and then paint the animal's name or message on it.
- Parents can take children to a garden centre and together select bulbs, plants or even trees for planting around the grave.

Cremation

After an animal has been cremated, children can help with decisions about the ashes. (They might not be prepared to touch or even look at them. It is even distressing for some adults to accept that these are all that is left of a good friend.)

- Ashes can be kept in a special casket and/or buried and the spot marked in some way.
- Ashes can be scattered on favourite walks and special places in the garden.
- Whatever the animal was, dog, mouse or fish, some sort of ritual is helpful. It is a way of showing respect, and the start of letting go.
- It is also an opportunity for the family to share the loss together and maybe talk about their feelings.

Memorials

Children can be encouraged to remember their animals and celebrate their lives by

- Writing poems or letters to the animal.
- Painting pictures.
- Making a scrap book with photographs and other reminders (pedigree, prize certificates from shows, bits of fur, etc.).

OTHER FACTORS WHICH INFLUENCE CHILDREN'S REACTIONS TO DEATH

- The honesty, sensitivity and understanding shown to children in connection with the loss of a treasured pet may not only help them deal with that loss, but also be a good preparation for dealing with future losses. They may also learn to trust and share things with parents.

- Obviously if children are having other difficulties in their lives, a pet's death may be the last straw and particular care must be taken to understand their problems. Sometimes, the pet's death makes an opportunity for them to open up and talk about the other worries.
- Children who have lost a loved human may have found difficulty in accepting the reality of that loss and therefore are unable to grieve appropriately. A pet's death is more tangible, and grieving for a pet may help a child to open up and mourn for the lost human as well.
- The presence of other animals sometimes helps children grieve. They may be able to pour out their hearts to an animal while still holding back with their family.
- Children have said that getting another animal really helped. The timing of this is important, so that it does not appear that the dead animal is being replaced. The child should be involved in deciding when it is the right time and in choosing a new animal.

FOR VETS AND PARENTS

Dos and don'ts

Do
- Make sure the child does not hear about the death from someone else.
- Always be honest about the death.
- Encourage the child to talk about their pet.
- Try to understand the importance of the animal, and what the child has lost.
- Be prepared to talk about how the animal died, but do not include distressing details.
- If a child is grieving, it may be a good idea to inform their teacher, but important to be discreet; do not talk about it in front of other children.
- Share your own feelings of sadness with the child.
- Never try to minimize their grief ('do not worry, I'll get you another one').
- Help with some sort of ritual.
- Help them to express their emotions, and accept that it may not be in tears.

- Do be willing to let the child have another animal. When/if you do, make it clear that it is not a replacement.

Do not
- Do not lie to a child about what happened. Their imagination is worse than the truth.
- Do not try to protect children by excluding them when discussing options or decisions.
- Never take an animal to be euthanased without letting the child know and say goodbye
- Do not remove the pet's belongings (leave that up to the child).
- Never underestimate their feelings.
- Do not trivialize the death ('after all, it is only a rat').
- Do not try to divert their grief ('Cheer up, I'll take you to McDonald's').
- Do not rush to get another animal immediately.
- Do not be afraid to admit your own feelings.
- Do not refuse to get another animal because of fears about a child's possible future grief.

Comments

Children have said that the following had made it more difficult for them:

- Not having any control or say in decisions about their pet.
- Lack of understanding from parents, friends, vets.
- No acknowledgement of their wishes or regrets.
- Not being prepared for the pet's death.
- Not having said goodbye.
- Not being allowed to stay with the animal at death (euthanasia).
- Not being able to take the body home.
- Not being allowed to have another animal.

See also Appendix 3–Books for Children

2

Getting a new animal

Returning to an empty home is always hard and those who have several animals know what a comfort the continuity of dog or cat presence can be. The greatest help in getting over the loss comes when we can bring ourselves to fill the gap again with a carefully chosen companion. Many people want to get another animal very soon, not being able to bear emptiness. They do not feel they are replacing their dead friend, but are replacing the 'dogness'/'catness' – that presence which helps to bring back some of the colour to their lives. However, when people are feeling sad over a death or loss, the time may not be right for the owner to embark on a new relationship and well-meaning people forget this. One family member may be longing for a dog or cat, but find that other members of the household are not yet ready for another.

There are many possible reasons why the idea of getting another animal is not appropriate yet for the owner.

- It is too soon. The final task of grieving is to be able to reinvest love in another. If there has been no deep grief, only sadness, then this may be accomplished in a few days. For those who are greatly troubled, then they need to 'process' their grief and they are the only ones who really can sense when the appropriate time is approaching. **Warning!** Urging someone to think about getting another animal may be unintentionally negating the depth of distress a person is feeling, when what is really needed at that time is an understanding of how painful and tough the situation is.
- The other side of that warning is that some grieving owners who really do want to get another pet might feel that people would think they never really cared enough for the dead one.
- Some people feel that they are betraying the love and affection of their dead pet if they decide to take on another animal.
- Occasionally people get trapped in their pain and cannot move on. In many cases, the misery of the death and pain of grief has been so disturbing (often unexpectedly so) that people are afraid

of being so hurt again. 'I'll never get another cat. It was like a long nightmare, I cannot go through that again.' When asked, 'Would you rather that you never had (Toby) in the first place? Was the joy he gave you not worth the suffering you went through?' most would say it was worth it, and they would go through anything to have had that animal.

All these reasons can be worked through at the right time if there is really a basic desire to have another animal.
There are other reasons of a more practical nature why people are hesitant about bringing in another animal.

- **Decreasing fitness or increasing debility of the person.** When the animal and person have been together for a long time, often their lifestyles and needs become much the same. They get to know each other so well and live in a comfortable harmony.
- If the animal dies, the person might very much want another animal, but may not feel able to cope with a whole new relationship, with possible problem behaviours or needs that would be difficult to cope with.
- It may be that they could adopt an older animal or maybe have another less demanding type of animal. Animal shelters and some vet practices will act as liaison for animals needing homes and those wanting animals. Some practices have small animal sanctuaries for unwanted pets.
- **Changed circumstances.** People may want another, but may be unable because they may not have complete autonomy in their own affairs. They may live with relatives or in a housing authority that allowed the old animal but refused permission to have another. This can be experienced as a great deprivation and it may be worth exploring alternatives. Financial circumstances such as vet bills can become too much for those with changed income circumstances.
- **People appreciating more freedom.** People who have been tied down to a certain extent by responsibilities to growing families, and later to a lesser extent by having to care for animals, may actually decide not to get another animal in the meantime, but take advantage of the freedom to travel and go away more than they had been able to do. They should not feel criticized for this decision.
- Many of the people approaching Rescue Centres have recently lost a pet and are seeking to replace it. They often need to talk about the one that they have lost and it is important to try and judge whether they are really ready for another pet. If this is done

too hastily the pet is returned because they are not ready to love another one, or it does not do what the other pet did. This leaves the person with another guilt factor and the animal with another rejection.

THE CHOICE

Apart from a strong breed preference, a new animal should not be selected because it looks like the previous one. This puts unreal expectations on an entirely different creature which should be appreciated for itself, not as a substitute. If they want the same breed, suggest they get a different colour.

When a new animal is chosen to join the household, the owner needs to be prepared for the completely different experience that relationship will bring. A whole new friendship will need to develop and it may take time.

It may sound strange but some people have found it useful to talk to the new animal about the old one, as a way of bridging the transition between them. One old man was heard saying to his new pup, 'Well, wee one, I know you are not Archie, and I cannot expect you to be, but you and I will grow to be pals too. And when you're bigger, I'll take you to the place he used to love.'

Things to avoid

- Do not talk about getting another animal when a person has just lost one that they loved a lot.
- Never suggest to a person that they might **replace** a dead animal.
- Do not surprise a grieving person with a new animal.
- Do not assume that someone did not love their dead animal if they get another right away.
- Do not assume that someone did not love their animal if they do not get another and decide they would rather not have that responsibility for a while.

Things you can suggest to a bereaved pet owner

- Do not be in a hurry to get another animal if you feel it is not the right time.
- Do be willing to allow yourself to get another animal if you have a feeling that you would really like to have an animal around again.

- You are not replacing any member of your pet family by getting a new one. What you are doing is positive and appropriate.
- Do not expect the new animal to be like the old one; be aware of the differences between young and mature animals.
- Do not expect to bond with a new animal right away.
- If someone has brought in a new animal, and you cannot get fond of it, do not feel you have to love it, but try to be reasonably kind. It is probably feeling lonely and rejected. Gradually, without pressure, you may grow fond of it.

3

Missing animals

When animals go missing, those responsible often become frantic with worry. All the worst scenarios are imagined. The emotions people feel are anxiety, fear, guilt and anger at themselves and others who may have been partly responsible. They are restless and cannot settle, often wandering around for hours searching for the lost pet.

Owners should:

- Check all sheds and buildings where an animal may have been shut in.
- Contact local police
- Phone or visit animal shelters and rescue centres, and if it is a dog, contact the dog wardens.
- Put adverts with description or pictures in local newspapers.
- Put up notices, with pictures, in local pet shops, supermarkets, the corner shop or local Post Office – these are likely to be attended by the local 'gossips' who have local knowledge!
- Phone neighbours. Ask them to look in sheds and outhouses.
- Phone up vet surgeries, in case an injured animal has been picked up.
- Put up notices in local vet surgeries. Make sure the date is on them. Let the vet know if the animal has been found.
- Phone the cleansing departments to check if the animal was killed on the road; leave a description.
- Alert delivery people, paper boys and girls, and the postman.
- If fitted with a microchip, ensure the company has your current address of owner.
- Notify the Lost Dog register.
- Some local radios have a lost and found slot that could be used.

If owners find pets, they should inform everyone who was looking and take down all the notices; otherwise they will interfere with any other searches for lost pets.

Waiting can be the hardest bit. Moments of hope alternate with fear. People may have difficulty sleeping, lying there wondering what has happened. Until an animal has been found, alive or dead, it is hard to know when to stop searching. The worry has no end, the grief no closure. As long as there is a chance of it being alive, the task of mourning cannot be completed.

The reality is that many missing animals, especially cats, do survive and may return home after several weeks, even months later. Many animals somehow end up in new homes, often having been taken in by people assuming they have been abandoned. (Occasionally cats will themselves adopt new owners.) These people may place adverts in the 'found' sections of local newspapers.

Some people have a fear about their animals having been 'sold for research'. They, however, can feel reassured because the law is very tight about this and no research establishment can use animals not especially bred for the purpose. If they were to do so, they would lose their licence to carry on their research.

For those who never do get reunited with their animals, there will probably always be seeds for worry somewhere, and maybe pangs of sadness and regret. Setting up or taking a role in a local Lost and Found service is a way that hard won experience may become of use to others.

4

Animals grieving for animals and animals grieving for humans

ANIMALS GRIEVING FOR ANIMALS

- When two or more animals have lived closely together for a long time, the loss of one individual might have some effect on the other(s).
- Owners may notice altered behaviour patterns and sometimes these may be similar to those of grieving humans (decreased appetite, changes in sleep patterns, unsettled, aimless wandering around, searching and crying, disinterest in other activities, loss of confidence, need for attention, and a general appearance of sadness).
- In many cases where the mutual attachment was not so strong, or when animals are more owner-orientated, surviving animals may not seem to be missing the dead one at all.
- They may be affected by the death through sensitivity to their owners' sadness as well as changes to their habitual routines.
- A very strong bond may develop between litter mates, if they have always been together.
- When several cats belong to one household, some of these may bond and interact closely. More often they may tolerate each other and tend to avoid interactions. When one of them dies, the surviving cat may behave differently. A cat that previously was shy, may come forward for attention. It may be lonely and missing the companionship. However, it might have been inhibited by the other, and now has more opportunity to be interactive and responsive.
- When one member of a social group dies, there may be a period of adjustment, with a rearrangement of positions. This particularly is the case if the one that died was the dominant dog in the pack. There may be temporary skirmishes and jostling for position.
- Pets' reactions to another pet's death vary enormously.
- To help pets cope with the death of a companion, it is usually a good idea to let them see the dead body, if possible before it has

gone cold. This may stop them searching and waiting anxiously for the return which will never happen.

- It is probably best not to let 'digging' dogs see where their friend is buried.
- It would appear that in some cases a temporary change of environment might reduce the impact of the severing of a long-term attachment.
- Other animals that are already present often help. If there are none, and death is foreseen, it may be useful to introduce another younger animal into the household before the death. The healthy animal will then have an opportunity to build up a new relationship, which may break, or reduce, the complete dependence on the dying animal. (The same holds true for humans who are totally involved with one animal, when it helps to get another before the death, as long as the older animal is able to cope.)
- When dogs are pining and grieving for a lost companion, getting another dog or even a cat is sometimes helpful. Do not expect it to be an immediate success. It takes time, at least a week or more for both to adjust and start building a new relationship as well. It should not be rushed.
- Bringing a new young animal is more successful with dogs than cats. Cats being more territorial, they often resent new strange cats, may never accept them as close companions, may completely ignore them, or even remain permanently hostile and aggressive.
- If death is expected for one of a close pair, it may be useful to feed them separately at different times, so that the surviving animal has become used to feeding alone.

ANIMALS GRIEVING FOR HUMANS

Animals that have for years shared the life of a human companion may show signs of grieving when their owner dies. As well as the behaviours mentioned in the previous section, there are some reports of pets dying 'of grief' following the death of a 'master'. The pattern is that of reactive depression and separation anxiety, which leads to stress, general anxiety and even death. This rarely happens, however, as most gradually adapt to an altered life, with a new focus for affection.

There are classic stories of faithful dogs who frequent the graves of their deceased owners; Greyfriars Bobby, whose statue stands near Greyfriars Church in Edinburgh, is a well-known Scottish one.

Whether or not an animal will adapt to life without its owner would depend on many things:

- The age of the animal.
- The length of the relationship.
- If it has been used to living with other people.
- Its basic nature (easy going or anxious).
- Whether or not the environment has changed.
- Keeping routines as normal as possible helps.

Cats that have become strongly bonded to one person over the years may have great difficulty adjusting to the loss of the person. They may hide, refuse food, resist handling (trying to escape) or become lethargic and apathetic. They may have dilated pupils and may fail to groom themselves. These behaviours and signs may continue for several weeks.

Some cats do adjust to a new home and to new people in a very short time. Owners should put the new address on the cat's collar. It is always advisable to keep them confined in their new surroundings for at least a week to make sure that they are eating well, before allowing them out. It is helpful to acquaint cats with the new neighbourhood by carrying them about (with a leash and harness, or in a wire basket) so that they can get their bearings before being out on their own.

Dogs, especially young ones, are more adaptable than cats, and usually will adjust to a new family and lifestyle in a short time.

When grieving animals are not eating well, it is important to try and get them eating again, but if they are constantly offered treats and special foods, they may develop into very fussy eaters so **care** must be taken with enticements.

What is the right thing to say when a friend's pet dies?

The fact that you are concerned enough to ask the question, probably means that you will do the right thing anyway – approach the friend and be there for them. Sometimes those who are bereaved have the distressing experience of feeling shunned by people who would normally be friendly. There appears to be such embarrassment and difficulty in confronting grief, that avoidance seems an easier option (but so hurtful to those already so lonely and vulnerable).

So, the most important thing is to be available, to listen, and be prepared to hear the same story over and over again. Talking is cathartic and can be encouraged by your attention and empathy. If asked, you can share a little of your own experiences, but avoid lengthy descriptions of your own personal bereavements. The time should be for them and your attention on their story, not on yours. Sometimes you might feel like saying, 'Do not worry, it will get better soon' or 'Time is a great healer', but this is not always helpful. We all know that things pass but somehow when we are really hurting, it is almost like hearing 'never mind'. We **do** mind and we need our suffering to be acknowledged, not diminished or minimised by someone trying to cheer us up.

No two situations are the same. Each relationship that has ended is unique and each one of us differs in the way we handle grief. Some people just do not want to talk about it and that must be respected. In some cases a statement like 'I guess you've been having a rough time' may be all that is needed to indicate your caring, with nothing more said. Sometimes a hug can be appropriate, and occasionally someone will want to let loose and sob in your arms. You just have to 'play it by ear' and get attuned to each one's special needs.

If your friend is feeling guilty, you can be reassuring that this is a problem particularly common for pet owners. Being so totally responsible for their animals during life, they take on the responsibility (and guilt) for the death as well. No matter what was done or was not done, people still manage to blame themselves for something. The 'IF ONLY' sometimes stands in the way of accepting the death, as if they could change the end of the story by a rerunning of events, over and over again.

Anger is also commonly experienced as part of grieving. It may be that someone deliberately did harm and the anger is therefore justified, but often there is an over-reaction to something which was done or said quite unintentionally. Anger may also be generalized about injustice or loss of belief. Acknowledging the anger and recognising the fact that it is frequently experienced after a bereavement, helps to keep it in perspective.

We suggest that all those who have had personal experience of the death of their own animals ask themselves: What was most helpful for me at the time? What should I have liked my friends to have said or done? What did I now want to hear? What was said or done that upset or angered me?

One thing that no pet owner would say, but others might, is 'Do not worry, you can get another one'. Though meant well, this feels like a total negation of the importance of the relationship that has just ended. However, the question sooner or later arises – 'What about another?'. Most of us for example, who love living with a dog, will have experienced the dreadful sense of emptiness in the home after a dog dies. Some need that gap filled as soon as the right dog can be found. This is in no way a replacement of the individual, but is a restoration of the 'dogness' in the home. Other people need time to adjust, to work through their grief before giving their love to a new pet.

They may feel guilty, believing that they are being disloyal by even thinking about getting another. It is as if letting go of their dead pet is implying that they could not have loved it so much; a sort of betrayal. It is almost as if hanging on to grief is necessary proof of our love. However, it does not have to be like that. We do not get over loving and missing those we have loved; we carry them in our hearts, as part of us. Nevertheless there is no rationing on love; we have unlimited capacities and though it may take time, we can allow ourselves to love again. It may be that grief has been so devastating that a person will say, 'No more, I cannot go through that again' and will deny themselves any future companionship with a pet. But the pain involved at parting is often the price we pay when someone has been important to us. Is the joy and friendship that a pet gives us not worth the suffering?

It is really a tribute to the memory of our dead friend that we are willing to take on a new relationship. Another pet reinstates the

PET presence, seeks your attention, demands to be fed and cared for, keeps you busy, and helps to abate the loneliness. Eventually, hopefully, it will work its way into your heart with its own special nature and gifts.

NOTES

Stress in veterinary practice

1

What are some of the stressors for vets in practice?

'Stress is when the perceived pressure on an individual exceeds that individual's ability to cope' or 'An excess of demands on an individual beyond their capability to cope'.

Stress, of course, is not always bad. A little stress can be good for us, keeping us stimulated, active and creative.

Some factors in life which affect stress

- Personal circumstances, finance, family, life transitions, state of health, etc.
- The type of job and position in that job.
- Relationships with other people.
- Expectations from others, and from oneself.
- Personality. High achievers and perfectionists (like many vets) are vulnerable.

STRESS IN VETERINARY PRACTICE

There are many stressors in the veterinary practice, particularly the high expectations of vets (from themselves as well as from their clients).

- Their student perceptions of being elite create a feeling of being 'different', even alienation.
- They are expected to be a credit to their profession, in manner, appearance and conduct.
- They must be good medics and surgeons and keep up with new developments and information.
- They are expected to be knowledgeable about the health and husbandry of every kind of animal.
- They are always expected to be respectful, considerate and courteous.
- They need to be competent at dealing with very emotional clients.

- They are expected to be caring and gentle with patients that may be aggressive and dangerous.
- They are regarded as educators, animal psychologists, rescuers.
- Sometimes they are expected to be surrogate social workers, counsellors, even undertakers.
- **And then they go home and face all the family generated expectations ...**

Professional stress

- Always having to be on top of things, sharp, intelligent and knowledgeable as well as skilful.

Business management stress

- Being practice owners and partners, worrying about finances and staff problems, when they want to be carrying out their professional work with their patients and clients.
- Having to keep financially afloat, as well as providing a caring service.

Loneliness

- After 5 years spent with fellow students in close relationships, going into practice can be extremely lonely. If the practice is small, vets are on their own with problem patients and clients.

Difficult clients

- Who assume more than is possible, expecting the vet to 'work miracles' for their animals.
- Who assume their vet will always be available to them at any hour of the day and night.
- Who may show disregard for their animals, or have neglected or abused them.
- Who may have personality problems that make them difficult to cope with.

Physical stress

- Long and uncertain hours.
- Overload of work, night calls, emergencies.
- Inability to say 'I am unwell'.

Emotional stress of dealing constantly with death and dying

- Having to cope with the emotions of clients and staff, as well as themselves.
- Having to be prepared for the emotional roller coaster of the work, going from death, to young healthy joyful animals, to euthanasia, etc. Having to adapt appropriate moods and behaviours.

Moral stress

- Being constantly faced with difficult ethical decisions.
- Killing healthy animals. (This is especially difficult for vets working in shelters.)
- Client's wishes and needs conflict with what is in the patient's best interests.

Staff problem

- Poor attitudes, poor morale, low motivation, squabbling, etc.

Being out of control

- The practice taking over all aspects of life.
- Being and feeling out of control is a primary cause of overstress.

2

Managing stress

RECOGNIZE THE SIGNS OF STRESS

- **Physical signs:** tiredness, headache, backache, tension, sleeping and digestive disorders, high blood pressure, all may contribute to heart disease, strokes, auto-immune disorders.
- **Emotional signs:** being bad tempered, anxious, grouchy, depressed, apathetic, defensive, ineffective, weepy, obsessed, critical, fearful, nervous.
- **Behavioural signs:** change in appetite, withdrawal from social contact, loss of judgement, forgetfulness, increased use of smoking, drink, drugs.

STRESS

- Lowers confidence and self-esteem.
- Lowers resistance to disease.
- Makes people prone to accidents.
- Increases the incidence of making mistakes.
- Causes breakdown in relationships.
- Creates more stress, and it keeps on escalating.
- Chronic persistent stress leads to 'burn-out', exhaustion and depression.

IDENTIFY THE STRESSES WHICH AFFECT YOU MOST

Make a list.

- Day to day stress – 'Oh, no – it is Monday again'; what is it about Mondays?

- Situation stress – think of your feelings when you are really stressed; then identify the source of those feelings. What situations, what people stress you most? Euthanasias? Business tasks? Emotional clients?
- Life stress. Living by someone else's rules; 'I should', 'I must'; fear of what might happen if . . .

Take steps to try and change things which can be changed. Be realistic about how much you can do. You cannot work miracles. You can do your best to facilitate a return to health where possible, but you cannot cure everything.

Be realistic about how much you should do. You are not omnipotent!

- Establish professional and personal boundaries appropriate for yourself
- Recognize that your boundaries may be different from other people's and respect both.

Learn to communicate effectively with your clients:

- Then you can enjoy your practice, and really value your clients and their pets.
- If a client is really dissatisfied, say confidently that there seems to be a lack of trust and if they would be happier in another practice you will send their case notes on to the vet they choose.

Delegate!

- Delegate everything that can be done by other staff, but do not overburden them.
- Encourage staff to do some training that will help them in dealing with clients (communication skills, bereavement support).

TIME MANAGEMENT

- Allow enough time for adequate consultation. Book a double slot for clients you know to be needing more time. 'Practices which allow consultation periods of up to 20–30 minutes per patient are more profitable, have happier clients, and have more satisfied vets and staff' (Dr Marty Becker, BSAVA Congress 1997). This is probably quite unrealistic for most vets to consider, but it is worth thinking about.

- If you and your staff learn to communicate effectively, you will all save time by not having to deal with misunderstandings, complaints and dissatisfied clients.
- Work out a reasonable rota for free time and keep to it if possible, keeping your private time private.
- Do not give out your home phone unless you do not mind being called.
- Always be sure that adequate emergency cover is available to your clients, so you do not feel guilty.
- Get away for complete breaks.

STAFF PROBLEMS

- Treat staff as equals. You are a team and no-one can function in isolation.
- Listen to the staff; they may be feeling emotionally stressed by the deaths they have to deal with.
- Have regular democratic staff meetings once a month, where everyone can air their feelings equally.
- Be able to exert authority but do not be unreasonable.
- Be willing to discuss with staff practice matters that have directly affected them. Feeling disempowered is a strong recipe for discontent. Get agreement where possible on staff policies.
- Be considerate of staff, be aware of their needs, and **acknowledge good effort and work.**
- Encourage staff motivation by extra training to expand capabilities and give them responsibilities.
- Encourage a member of staff to attend a course on support for grieving clients. This will give them confidence, as well as taking some of the total burden from you.
- Arrange staff social evenings so that all the staff can relax and have some fun together. Some practices find that going out once a month together (bowling, go-carting, racing, swimming) builds a sense of camaraderie that is extremely beneficial to the practice as a whole.

ANXIOUS CLIENTS

Instead of being hounded by clients phoning in with queries about in-patients or lab reports, sometimes a policy of 'get them before they get to you' works well. A system of proactive telephone calls allows you to phone at your convenience and can take place before the client feels the need to phone.

PATIENT PROBLEMS

A vet writes:

One of my biggest stresses is related to patients with problems that I've either not solved or resolved. I find referring to someone else for a second opinion, be it on an ECG, X-ray or the whole case, is an enormous help. Conferring with someone else helps spread the load, and relieve the pressure.

MORAL STRESS ASSOCIATED WITH UNNECESSARY KILLING OR CONFLICTING ISSUES

- This is never easy; there may be no satisfactory answer.
- Moral stress affects people differently according to their personal standards and ethical opinions.
- Establish a practice policy that sets out guidelines for ethical practice, but be prepared to be flexible as appropriate.
- If you are employed in a practice with ethical guidelines that conflict with your own and you are unable to influence things, it is best to look for a practice where you will feel more at ease.
- Personal stress can be lowered by feeling that you have done your best to alleviate the problem in individual cases and to make some sort of contribution in general situations (see Section 2.1).

EMOTIONAL STRESS ASSOCIATED WITH ANIMAL DEATH, EUTHANASIA AND DISTRESSED CLIENTS

- This is potentially the greatest source of stress in practice for the vets and the nurses.
- If handled well it can also be the greatest source of satisfaction and the aspect of your work that is most appreciated by your clients.

When things cannot be changed, keep a sense of humour. Increase your ability to cope. Be kind to yourself: do not ignore your emotional and physical needs.

Look after your physical needs

- Get enough sleep. Eight hours sleep is best for optimum health and efficient work.
- Exercise regularly (even if you are tired); even as little as 20 minutes hard exercise several times a week is beneficial.
- Eat well, lots of fruit and vegetables.
- Learn to relax; if you cannot, take time to go on a course or read up on relaxation techniques.

Look after your emotional and social needs

- Try to have some fun; develop an interest in something not associated with work.
- Be an active member of your community in some way that appeals to you.
- Try to have some sort of mutual personal support system with a friend (not a partner).
- Keep work worries and family life separate if possible.
- Seek help if things get beyond you. Your medical practice may have a counsellor you can consult.
- If you are interested in Human Animal Bond work, you can establish links with community carers and social workers, psychiatric nurses, etc. You can help them out with establishing pet therapy programmes, or pet fostering and they might give you support and advice with personal or work-related issues, or with difficult client situations.
- Contact specific services set up for the support and help of members of the veterinary profession.

Do not expect miracles from yourself

- Just try your best; then acknowledge to yourself that you are doing your best. No one is perfect.
- Share responsibilities. Have regular weekly meetings with colleagues to discuss casework, and bounce ideas, and share feelings about cases.

As you start coping better and are not so severely stressed, you become more effective in changing potentially stressful situations!

The 'vicious circle' works in reverse!

If you always do what you've always did,
you'll always get what you always got!
Try something different
(Anon)

Veterinary nurses' perspectives

The nurses have differing roles and responsibilities, and are crucial in the smooth and pleasant running of the practice.

As well as clinical nursing duties, they are also expected to provide emotional and psychological support both to the patients and clients. They are usually the ones who have to spend time listening to clients' anxieties and complaints, and to be supportive while always remaining loyal to the practice.

If the practice has a hospital and keeps in-patients, then the nurses will probably become more bonded to the animals and more emotionally involved in each situation than the vets will.

THINGS WHICH ARE A SOURCE OF SADNESS

Sadness for the animals

Through the nursing and caring, nurses get genuinely fond of some animals, and are upset when their condition worsens and they die or must be euthanased.

Sadness for the grief of others

The distress of owners especially affects nurses when the client is a friend, is lonely or disadvantaged, but most sadness is felt for elderly people strongly bonded to their pets. It is appropriate for nurses to let owners know that they feel sad as well, but it is also important that they do not keep holding on to the sadness after the people have left, and they have new challenges to face.

Things which are a source of anger or frustration

Clients

- Clients with a casual attitude towards life, who bring in healthy animals for destruction, for trivial reasons.

- Clients who have neglected or abused their animals.
- Clients who do not consider that any other animals matter except theirs, and are excessively demanding.
- Clients who are abusive or blame them unjustly.

Vets
- Who seem off-hand and clumsy, even callous in dealings with clients and patients.
- Who have not taken time to explain things or prepare clients for possible poor outlooks.
- Who have given clients false optimism.
- Who have pressurised clients into decisions before adequate discussion of options.
- Whose scientific curiosity, or financial interests may influence a choice of action questionable for the welfare of the animal.
- Who do not seem to care about or take an interest in the animal for itself, only as a case.
- Who leave them to deal with the task of chasing up reports and explaining delays or problems to anxious owners.
- Who take for granted all the effort they put in, never acknowledge them or say thanks.
- Who do not acknowledge their feelings.
- Who pile on extra work clearing up after them, never offering to help even when they have free time.
- Who do not support them when clients complain about them unjustly.

Colleagues
- Who do not care enough about the animals, or people.
- Who do not seem to notice when they are over-stretched or exhausted and do not help.

Things which can be a source of guilt

Nurses often seem to take on guilt in a lot of situations where they have been involved, but obviously have not been responsible for things out of their control, such as:

- When anything goes wrong in the practice.
- Deterioration of condition or death in animals they have been caring for.
- Euthanasia of healthy animals under anaesthesia, especially when in for optional procedures.
- Having to tell owners bad news.

Things that help to make the practice a good place to work

- Keeping a sense of humour.
- The animals in general. Seeing the vets spend time being with and talking to the animals.
- Working with vets who are kind to their clients and patients.
- Seeing animals getting better, especially when they have been hospitalized.
- Seeing shy, nervous animals get confident and have trust in them (especially in-patients).
- Good team work. People helping each other out, including the vets, when things are busy.
- Improved communication. People asking for, and listening to, each other's ideas and concerns. Vets communicating with clients so there are no misunderstandings.
- Sharing emotional upsets with other staff (staff meeting where everyone has equal say).
- Being encouraged and given opportunities to learn more and do more; going on courses.
- Feeling that they are appreciated, and their contribution to the practice is acknowledged.
- Receiving photos of previous patients looking well and healthy.
- Getting appreciative letters from owners.

Summary information

Complaints

The majority of complaints received by The Royal College of Veterinary Surgeons deal with negligence and misdiagnosis/treatment of animals AND the mistreatment of clients.

- **The RCVS.** Many complaints to The Royal College would appear to have arisen because of poor communication/misunderstanding with the client and, in some cases, rudeness. There are some veterinary surgeons who do not appreciate that they are treating the client as well as the animal, or do not care about the client.
- **The Veterinary Defence Society** reports that the majority of cases which end up in the Small Claims Court could have been avoided if a veterinary surgeon had had better communication skills.
- **The Pet Bereavement Support Service** volunteers accept anonymous calls from people distressed by the death of a pet. Often the grief has been exacerbated by actions taken or not taken by the veterinarians involved. The veterinary surgeons are never identified and the observations, sometimes complaints, are very seldom formally reported. The callers' concerns about their veterinary surgeon provide a valuable source of information by revealing the types of situation, actions and attitudes that upset owners, which make it even more difficult to come to terms with their sorrow or grief.

WHAT DO CLIENTS COMPLAIN ABOUT?

Diagnosis/treatment

Persistent confusion about the diagnosis and treatment
- The diagnosis was not satisfactorily explained to them, they did not understand what it meant or why it took so long to reach, resulting in lack of confidence in the veterinary surgeon.

- They were given the impression that certain expensive treatments would prolong their animals' lives when in fact their animals died soon after treatment began.

Multiple veterinary surgeons
- Clients were concerned at apparent lack of continuity of attending veterinarians or that their animals were nervous of certain veterinary surgeons.
- Lack of confidence in their skill, interest and familiarity with the case.

Veterinary surgeons were un-cooperative, rude or angry
In cases when asked to:

- Make a home visit.
- Perform euthanasia at home.
- Arrange for a second opinion.
- Arrange for a consultation with a veterinary surgeon who practised complementary medicine.

Refusal to make home visits, refusal to attend emergencies
- Many complaints were about death following the refusal of veterinary surgeons to attend an emergency call.
- Veterinarians were rude or abusive as well as refusing to attend.
- Veterinary surgeons had no apparent emergency cover for their practice.

Attitude of veterinary surgeons towards them or their animals
- Veterinarian perceived as being indifferent – callous, uncaring.
- Unfamiliar veterinary surgeons attending the case, with no obvious knowledge of the history or concern for the animal.

Euthanasia/follow-up

Unsatisfactory help with decisions – clients
- Felt that the veterinary surgeon was unwilling or angry when asked to perform euthanasia at home, failing to explain why it was in the animal's interest for it to be performed in the surgery.
- Felt that they may have waited too long, causing the animal to suffer.
- Did not understand the reason for euthanasia; felt it might have been unnecessary or premature.
- Felt they had been pressurised or persuaded into euthanasia with no opportunity for discussion.

At euthanasia (client present)
- Veterinary surgeon handled animal roughly; did not seem to care that they were killing a much-loved pet.
- Euthanasia being, or appearing to be, painful and traumatic for the animal.
- Difficulty in injecting a struggling, frightened animal.
- Changing injection sites and going into the body cavity or organs.
- Dogs being muzzled while dying.

Animals euthanased without owner's permission, brought in by someone else – clients not being present at their animal's death
- Animal dying after being admitted for treatment or surgery, with no opportunity to say goodbye.
- Owner unprepared for animal's possible death; upset that it died alone.
- Owner upset that they were told the news over the telephone, in an unsympathetic manner, or did not learn of the death until arriving to collect the animal.

Misunderstandings about the options for disposal of the animal
- Not enough discussion beforehand about the options available.
- Uncaring voice when told the ashes were ready; unsympathetic reception when collecting ashes.

Inappropriate handling of the body
- Bodies not treated with respect; owners witnessing bodies put into body bags.
- Bodies handed back to owners in dishevelled state, heads hanging down and tongues lolling out, still bloody after unsuccessful operation or even with wound still unclosed.

Veterinary surgeons not available or approachable for answering questions or giving reassurance after death
- When there had not been enough opportunity for questions before death, owners were left with grave doubts which needed to be addressed.

Other complaints made officially

- Veterinary surgeons have been perceived as being rude, uncaring and disinterested.

- Veterinary surgeons have been unsympathetic, cold and callous when animal very ill or dying.
- Veterinary surgeons abusive to the animal and client, careless or rough in handling animal.
- Holding back information, even deceiving owner.

2

Things clients are grateful for

ATTITUDES OF THE VET AND ALL THE STAFF

- A warm reception and friendly attitude.
- Recognizing the owner and the animal, especially remembering the animal's name.
- Taking an interest in the owner and the animal.
- Showing respect, making the client feel confident.
- Being aware of difficult situations, and reacting kindly and being supportive.

HANDLING THE ANIMAL

- The vets and staff taking great pains to make the animal feel relaxed and comfortable.
- Speaking to the animal, using its name, being kind and gentle.
- Making appreciative comments, letting the owner know that the animal is liked and valued.

THE NURSES' CARE AND KIND ATTENTION, ESPECIALLY IF ANIMALS ARE ADMITTED

Being a 'good' vet including being attentive, interested and caring. Taking the time and making an effort.

- Explaining everything that is being found, that is being considered.
- Discussing things, listening, encouraging questions, ensuring understanding.
- Being honest.
- Being understanding and compassionate.
- Being kind, strong, confident and in control.

- Managing euthanasia in a caring sensitive way.
- Giving the animal a peaceful 'good death'.
- Being supportive to the client all the way through.
- Allowing the client as much time with the deceased pet as they need.
- Arranging privacy for distressed clients.
- Sending 'condolence' cards or personal letters.

All that has been recommended in the previous sections as being good practice, has in one way or another been mentioned by clients as having been appreciated.

Possible consequences of poor management

EFFECT ON CLIENTS

- They may be angry, troublesome, 'difficult', even abusive to staff and vets.
- They may be unhappy, guilty, depressed and stuck in their grieving.
- They will undoubtedly tell all their family and friends about their grievances.
- They may feel unable to get another pet because of what happened.
- They may want to 'take the matter further'.

EFFECT ON THE VETS

- Anger, feeling persecuted, misunderstood.
- Feeling guilty, sad, embarrassed.
- Low self-esteem, self-doubt, feeling incompetent.
- Dread of repeats (like difficult euthanasias).
- Angst, stress, tension.
- Feelings of failure.
- Loss of professional satisfaction.

EFFECT ON VETERINARY STAFF

- Low morale.
- Feeling embarrassed.
- General tension.
- Strained relationships: grumpy or crabby colleagues, angry boss.
- Lack of pleasure.
- Feeling sad for clients, animals.

EFFECT ON PRACTICE REPUTATION AND PERSONAL REPUTATION

- Locally: bad news travels fast, and the practices soon get unfavourable reputations.
- Professionally, the vets may be called up to the disciplinary committee of the RCVS. Their names are published in the report, even when they have been cleared of the charge. All the veterinary community is aware. Their names may be temporarily removed from the register. In the cases of gross misconduct they may be 'struck off'. If they are taken to court, their names may be made public.

EFFECT ON THE PROSPERITY OF THE PRACTICE

- The aggrieved clients may not return.
- If they get another animal they will register with another practice.
- New clients asking around may be dissuaded from attending that practice.
- The practice may not prosper.

4

Possible consequences of good management

EFFECTS ON CLIENTS

- Feeling supported and understood and grateful to vets and staff.
- Reassured that everything was done that could have been done.
- Confident that decisions were made correctly.
- Not feeling angry and guilty, but able to get on with their grieving or sorrowing.
- Not left with unfinished business.
- Likely to get another animal at some point.
- Remaining loyal to the practice.

REASONS GIVEN FOR CHOICE OF VET

In a study done in USA it was found that, apart from locality, vets were selected because of (1) their character; (2) their way of handling the animal; (3) their ability to communicate and (4) (and last) their professional skills.

EFFECT ON THE VETS

- Feelings of job satisfaction.
- Personal satisfaction.
- Self-confidence.
- Enjoyment.
- Good relationships with others.

BASIC HUMAN NEEDS

- There is need for **shelter**, **physiological needs** of food, clothing, etc. Vets obviously have to provide for these by running a successful business.
- People also need **recognition**, **appreciation**, **acceptance** and **affiliation**.
- Vets who get the reputation of being caring and understanding and willing to take a role in the community can partly fulfil these needs through their relationships with their clients and the community.
- Another basic need everyone has is **to fulfil whatever potential is there**, and if vets have a thriving practice and an appreciative clientele, they are more likely to have the opportunity of striving to be a successful vet and to enjoy their professional life.

EFFECTS ON THE STAFF

- There is more recognition of everyone's importance as part of a team.
- The staff work hard and need to be appreciated, and thrive on it.
- Grateful clients stimulate great job satisfaction (they also bring gifts).
- The relationships amongst the staff are better.
- There is more efficiency and enthusiasm for work.

EFFECTS ON THE PRACTICE

- The practice will attract clients who have heard about its reputation.
- The practice will thrive.
- It will be a good place to work and to be associated with.

APPENDICES

Appendix 1

Rough guide to life spans – life expectancies of companion animals

Although owners want to know the expected life span of their particular type of pet, it is difficult to find an agreed consensus on the average life spans of many of our companion animals. The ages given below are only a rough guide. Some animals age much more quickly than others and some individuals live to extraordinary ages. Owners who have heard of such animals often expect theirs to be equally long lived.

Dogs	small hardy breeds 13–16+ (some to 20+ years)
	medium large dogs 11–13+ (giant breeds 8–10 years)
Cats	average life expectancy around 10–14+ years, may live to over 20!
Mice	1–2.5 years
Rats	2–3 years
Gerbils	1.5–3 years
Hamsters	1.5–2 years
Rabbits	male 8+ years/female 6+ years
Guinea pigs	4–7+ years
Ferrets	5–7+ years (up to 11)
Chinchillas	10–15 years
Chipmunks	male 3 years/female 5 years
Budgies	3–5+ years (not many reach more than 10–11, but have been reported as living up to 20)
Canaries	5–6+ years (exceptionally over 14)
Tortoises	possibilities of very long lifespans, up to 80+ years
Small lizards/snakes	3–10 years
Larger pythons/boas	can live up to 30+ years
Horses	can live till around 35+ years, but most are killed before they become geriatric
Donkeys	around 40+ years

Resources and useful addresses

Society for Companion Animal Studies (SCAS)
10(B) Leny Road
Callander
Perthshire FK17 8BA
Tel./Fax: 01877 330996
Can often help with identifying other addresses of national organizations. SCAS also provides a training video (*A Kind Goodbye*), a training/study manual (*When a Pet Dies*) and training sessions for veterinary practices on request.

'The Really Useful Address List' is updated annually and is available from:
Grayling
4 Bedford Square
London WC1B 3RA
Tel: 0171 255 1100
Contact national organizations to obtain details of local branches or services.

The Pet Bereavement Support Service
Tel. 0800 09 666 06
Is a nationwide telephone helpline for pet owners who are referred to a local befriender.

Appendix 3

Further reading

FOR VETERINARY PRACTITIONERS

AVMA Guidelines for Responding to Clients with Special Needs (1995), *Journal of the American Veterinary Medical Association*, vol. 206, no. 7, pp. 961–976.

Bower, J. (1997) *Veterinary Practice Management* (2nd edn). Blackwell, Oxford.

BVA (1989) *Killing with Kindness: Compassionate Euthanasia*, Proceedings of a BVA symposium. British Veterinary Association, London.

Cohen, S. and Fudin, C. (1991) *Problems in Veterinary Medicine – Animal illness and human emotion*, vol III, no.1. J. B. Lippincott Company, Philadelphia.

Fogle, B. and Abrahamson, D. (1990) Pet loss: a survey of the attitudes and feelings of practising veterinarians. *Anthrozoos*, vol. III, no. 3.

Kay, W. J. and Cohen, S. P. (eds) (1988) *Euthanasia of the Companion Animal*. The Charles Press, Philadelphia.

Lagoni, L., Butler, C. and Hetts, S. W. B. (1994) *The Human–Animal Bond and Grief*. Saunders, Philadelphia.

Lagoni, L. (1997) *The Practical Guide to Client Grief*. AAHA Press, Colorado.

BOOKS FOR GENERAL INFORMATION ON THE HUMAN–ANIMAL RELATIONSHIP

Beck, A. and Katcher, A. (1984) *Between Pets and People*. Perigree Books, New York.

Fogle, B. (ed.) (1981) *Interrelations between People and Pets*. C.C. Thomas, Springfield, Illinois.

Ironside, V. (1994) *Goodbye, Dear Friend*. Robson Books, London.

Katcher, A. and Beck, A. (eds.) (1983) *New Perspectives on our Lives with Companion Animals* (2nd edn). University of Philadelphia Press, Philadelphia.

Lee, M. and L. (1992) *Absent Friend*. Henston, High Wycombe.

Nicholson, J. (ed.) (1993) *Pet Loss and Support for Bereaved Pet Owners*. Report of a conference of the Society for Companion Animal Studies, Callander, Perthshire.

Robinson, I. (ed.) (1995) *The Waltham Book of Human–Animal Interactions*. Pergamon, Oxford.

Serpell, J. (1988) *In the Company of Animals*. Cambridge University Press, Cambridge.

Serpell, J. (ed.) (1988) *Companion Animals in Society*. Oxford University Press, Oxford.

BOOKS FOR CHILDREN

For young children

Large, C. (1996) *Bye Bye Belle*. Farewell Publishing, London.

Valey, S. (1985) *Badger's Parting Gifts*. Collins, Picture Lions Series, London.

Voist, J. (1971) *The Tenth Good Thing About Barney*. Collins, Glasgow.

Wilhelm, H. (1985) *I'll Always Love You*. Hodder & Stoughton, Sevenoaks, Kent.

For children over 8 years

Simmons, P. (1989) *Fred*. Young Puffin, London.

General

St Catherine's Hospice (1988) *A Child's Questions About Death*. St Catherine's Hospice, Crawley.

Index